From Cave to Computer

A New Perspective on
the Homeopathic Miasms

From Cave to Computer

A New Perspective on
the Homeopathic Miasms

Maria Jevtic

2012

ISBN 9781-874581-727   r0

Printed by Berforts Information Press Ltd, Stevenage, UK
Text and artwork © Winter Press, 2012
Published by Winter Press in 2012

Winter Press
16 Stambourne Way
West Wickham, Kent BR4 9NF
e: c2c@winterpress.net

"It has become appallingly obvious that our technology has exceeded our humanity"
Albert Einstein

Contents

About the Author xi

Acknowledgements xiii

Introduction 1

In Paradise 4

The Dawn of Spirituality — Did Early Humans get Sick?
— Susceptibility and Disease Stimulus — The Law of
Similars — Attitude, Behaviour and Chronic Disease — Psora
— Parasites

The Agricultural Revolution 25

Cereals — Acidity — Minerals and Vitamin B — Lectins
— Mould — Slowing Down — Addiction — Cereals and
Anxiety — Chronic Back-ground Anxiety — Disease Agents
— Exercise — The Shift from Acute to Chronic — Physical
Psora — Digestion — Liver and Kidney — Respiratory and
Skin — Allergy — Psoric Disease Stimuli — The Benefits of
Psora — Epigenetics — Up and Beyond Psora — The Story of
Chronic Disease in a Nutshell — Parallel to Psora

The Life Of A Nomad 54

Animal Husbandry — The Male Nomad — The Female Nomad
— Tubercular Attitude — Tuberculosis, the disease — Cross-
Infection — Dairy — Dairy Intolerance — Acidity — Mineral
Imbalances — Phosphorus and Vitamin D — Inflammation
and Arachidonic Acid — Allergy — Early Nomad's Disease
Process — Addiction and the Adrenal Glands — Physical
Tuberculosis — Summary of Tuberculosis — The Benefits of
Tuberculosis, the Miasm — Beyond Tuberculosis

Urbanisation 78

    To Have or To Have Not — Class Society — Urban Life — The
    Physical Disadvantages of Urban Life — Lack of Exercise —
    Yeast and Mould — Refined Grains, Blood Sugar and the
    Adrenal Glands — Sugar — Diet across the Classes — Sycotic
    Behaviour, or the Urban Female — Sycotic Attitude Married
    to Sycotic Stimulus — Urban Stress and Spirituality —
    Benefits of Sycosis — Recreational Drugs

Monotheism 105

    Confucianism — Sycosis and Syphilis – Two Sides of the Same
    Coin — Discipline — Perversion — Fear and the Adrenal
    Glands — Syphilis, Symmetry and the Immune System —
    Fasting and the Syphilitic Diet — Syphilis — Mercury — The
    Mercury Miasm — In the Wake of Syphilis, the Miasm — The
    Benefits of Syphilis

Globalisation. 134

    The Scientific Revolution — Globalisation and the Age of
    Reason — The Nature of Reason — Tolerance — All is One
    — A New Miasm — Cancer, the Ultimate Multi-factorial
    Problem — Emotional Suppression — Harmony, or the
    Susceptibility to Cancer — The Ethical Vegetarian — Trust
    versus Control — Disease in the Realm of Cancer — Auto-
    immunity — Toxic World - Toxic Body — Toxicity Quotes
    and Statistics — The Benefits of the Cancer Miasm

Conclusion. 192

    Maintaining Causes — Therapeutic Implications — A Cure

Appendix 1 — Cancer & Science 197

Appendix 2 — Practical Advice 201

Bibliography 203

About the Author

Born in Germany, Maria moved to the UK in 1986 to study violin and viola at the Guildhall School of Music and Drama in London. After finishing her performer's course she became a member of the orchestra of the Royal Opera House where she worked for 7 happy years.

Not entirely satisfied with her career as a musician, she left the orchestra and trained as a Nutritionist at the former Plaskett Nutritional Medicine College and later as a homeopath at the Centre for Homeopathic Education. She obtained her BSc Hons in 2008. Living and working in Wimbledon, she combines her private practice with her family life. Apart from her first book "DIY Health Guide", Maria has recently also begun publishing articles, giving health related talks and running an Arnica network group (www.arnica.org.uk).

Acknowledgements

The original idea for "From Cave to Computer" came to me after reading Loren Cordain's book "The Paleo Diet". After gradually changing my own way of eating to an approximation of Cordain's modern day hunter-gatherer diet, I began wondering whether Cordain's linking of chronic disease to the agricultural transition could indeed be translated into homeopathic terms. I sat down at my computer and explored the idea, beginning with Psora.

My association of Psora with settlers and Tuberculosis with nomads I would trace back to a book by Peter D'Adamo, who writes about the "blood type diet". Whilst I do not subscribe to the idea that our blood type determines healthy food choices, Adamo's division into hunters, settlers and nomads nevertheless let me believe that at least in a purely schematized way, there could indeed be a link to chronic disease and its evolution.

Much of the nutritional evidence required for this book had already been gathered during my studies and practice as a qualified nutritionist, and it just needed to be put in order. The information about early humans, first settlements, urban life, world religions etc is either part of my general knowledge, or was found accidentally whilst reading seemingly unrelated material. Occasionally, I conducted careful internet searches of scientific literature.

As I reached the end of Psora, then Tuberculosis, I wondered whether the other miasms could also be explained or associated with similarly monumental changes in our way of life. As it turned out, the answer was "yes", and so I continued.

I would ask the reader to take this book as just one valid model for understanding miasms. As we know, what seems to be correct at one time, may turn out to be nonsense fifty years later. But interestingly, I found an emerging body of evidence showing that my thoughts were on the right track.[1]

In particular, an essay by Jared Diamond – scientist and author – added convincing support to the idea that all disease of body and mind and pretty much everything else that is wrong with society and how its individuals conduct themselves is due to the biggest error in human history: the first agricultural revolution.[2] I only found his article after I finished writing my book, but I am delighted to see that my ideas are in good company.

I also found encouragement in the fascinating home-opathic writings of Jeremy Sherr[3], Ian Watson[4], Colin Griffith[5] and Peter Fraser[6]. Again, I came to these while I was researching for support of my idea. Jeremy Sherr's

1   Robson AJ. A Bioeconomic View of the Neolithic Transition to Agriculture. Canadian Journal of Economics. 2010; 43(1):280-300
     Cohen MN and Armelagos GJ, eds. Paleopathology at the Origin of Agriculture. New York. 1994; Academic Press
     Steckel RH and Jerome C. The Backbone of History: Health and Nutrition in the Western Hemisphere. Cambridge. 2002; Cambridge University Press
2   Diamond J. The Worst Mistake in the History of the Human Race. Discover Magazine. 1987; pp. 64-66.
3   Sherr J. Organon as Light. The Homeopath, 2010; 111-115
4   Watson I. The Homeopathic Miasms, a Modern View. Totnes. 2009; Cutting Edge Publications
5   Griffith C. The Companion to Homeopathy. London. 2005; Watkins
6   Fraser P. Using Miasms in Homeopathy. West Wickham. 2008; Winter Press

essay "Organon as Light", in particular, seems to me to be expressing similar ideas to mine – although in a beautifully poetic way, only hinting at his true understanding.

To conclude, I am not aware of any work similar to my rather more factual view of the homeopathic miasms. I therefore hope that this will make it a valuable contribution to our understanding and approach to healing.

Introduction

As homeopaths we are interested in prevention and cure; not only of a particular ailment, but of chronic disease in general.

Hahnemann thought the existence of chronic disease to be due to miasms – without Psora, the original miasm, mankind would not suffer from chronic ailments. After Psora other miasms followed, but the idea remained the same – miasms were disease entities which deranged the vital force in such a way that self-guided recovery was impossible. Even the strictest living habits and the healthiest attitudes would not stop them from getting a hold on us and deranging our vital force for ever. Chronic disease would slowly but surely creep up on us and get us in the end.

Thankfully Hahnemann discovered a remedy. He found that giving anti-miasmatic homeopathic medicines would slow down or even reverse these evil influences and would help our vital force to resist. There was a cure after all. Or so he believed.

Nowadays, our experience is sobering. Rather than preventing chronic disease, homeopathy may only buy us time. Yes; we manage to cure a presenting complaint, but more often than not we see another one surfacing sooner or later. To be fair, a person undergoing extensive homeopathic treatment over many years, even if interrupted, generally moves in the right direction, i.e. from more serious to less serious complaints. But sometimes, and recently more often, we have seen homeopaths themselves falling victims to the deepest of chronic diseases.

In trying to find an explanation one could perhaps say that there might be fewer cases of deep disease amongst homeopaths than amongst the general population. However, we have no way of verifying this. Without wanting to point a finger, one might ask whether incorrect homeopathic treatment, suppression or unfavourable living habits are to blame. But on the whole, we can probably assume that it is neither a lack of expertise nor maturity that causes these very sad and sobering deaths.

So why, with all our knowledge and expertise, do we not get beyond buying time? Is it simply a case of old age? A case of having to die of something?

Is this just miasm at work? But if this is the answer, why do not our miasmatic nosodes and anti-miasmatic remedies at least prevent the worst and at best allow us to truly just die in our sleep? In most cases our remedies do not do this and so there must be something wrong with our theory or with our application of it. Or perhaps with our perception of chronic disease.

Keeping this in mind, perhaps it is time to take stock, to evaluate our methods and examine our understanding. Perhaps we are missing a vital piece in the puzzle of chronic disease. This piece of information may simply not have been available to Hahnemann and his early followers.

With extremes of environmental pollution on the one hand and an explosion of scientific and technological advances on the other, we have reached the age of globalisation and mutually shared information. As homeopaths, are we going to use these newly found insights to solve the puzzle of chronic disease? I believe we must.

The following is my view on chronic disease; its origins and its evolution through the ages, from cave to computer and beyond. All I ask of you, the reader, is to keep an open mind. This is because what follows may go beyond the comfortable.

In Paradise

In biblical paradise the world was in order, and harmony prevailed. Man had not become self-aware and had not acquired the knowledge of good and evil. The moment he did, disaster struck. Thus it seems that all our answers are in Genesis.

Non-biblical paradise, however, did not exist. Or did it?

More than 1.5 million years ago several hominid two-legged species lived side-by side in Africa. Their level of consciousness is not known. Their animal ancestors would definitely not have been self-aware to the degree that we are now, and they would not be able to see into the future beyond what was necessary for their survival. Getting worried about tomorrow or dwelling on yesterday would not be instrumental for the survival of the fittest. The zebra will not stop crossing the river just because it remembers from last month's crossing that there are crocodiles in it. It may be scared but it is programmed to override this fear, as it needs to get across to greener grazing grounds.

Similarly, applying good and evil, judgment and value to any animal actions would be nonsense as an animal's only guiding force is its instinct. You do not ask a lion to stop slaughtering baby antelopes because it seems a little cruel. Instinct programmes animals to do only what is good for the survival of the species.

Back to our hominids, these ancestors would have been very similar to animals, i.e. programmed for the survival of the species. But somewhere along the line they began changing outwardly as well as inwardly, slowly but surely moving away from their animal past into their human future.

At some time between 500,000 to 200,000 years ago they achieved the control of fire and most probably began cooking their food. In Europe and some parts of Asia and the Middle East, Neanderthal man roamed the wilderness. He was an apex predator, meaning he had no other creature above him in the food chain. Neanderthal lived almost exclusively on meat and his brain was larger than ours. But he was doomed as 190,000 years ago homo sapiens arrived on the evolutionary road. All of us are of this species, defined by our present brain size and the ability to make tools purposefully.

Homo sapiens crowded out all other species of hominids, but may have interbred with Neanderthal and perhaps others, as some believe.

50,000 years ago behavioural modernity and language was fully established. This meant that humans were conversing as well as engaging in spiritual and cultural practices. They were burying their dead and looking after their wounded.

Inwardly, this change was accompanied by an awakening of self-awareness, and with it an ability to make intellectual and emotional choices outside the bounds of instinct. Additionally man could now anticipate into the far future as well as dwell on the past. This had several consequences – a self-aware being was beginning to see himself as separate from others. He was not necessarily guided by the compulsion of his instincts to ensure the survival of the species, but he could now take action to preserve his own life before anyone else's. Additionally he was beginning to attach value to his actions, therefore bringing in ethical considerations. We can see that the awakening of self-awareness and intellectual choice brought with it a split; a split between himself and others, and the duality of good and evil.

Consider the following hypothetical event.

200,000 years ago, you are out hunting with your mates, about nine of you altogether. It is near dark and the sun is about to go down over the African horizon. Your best mate is injured and cannot make his way back to camp. The terrain is too rough to carry him and in any case carrying him would slow you down and you would not make it back to the safety of the camp where the rest of the clan are waiting for the game you hunted today.

A further couple of million years before this, as pack-hunting animal, you would have been compelled by your instinct to leave him to ensure the survival of the group. There was no programme for empathy over survival or even just for physically carrying an injured mate. Can you apply ethics to such a decision? Of course not. Animals are out of ethical bounds. The only thing that counts is the survival of the species, and all choices are based on this.

Additionally, the injured would – once deceased – supply the rest of nature with protein and minerals and thus provide the food chain with valuable ingredients: some animals would feed on the flesh, the bones would be crunched up, insects and worms and even bacteria and other single-celled organisms would finish off the rest. Ashes to ashes, dust to dust. The weakest are sacrificed for the benefit of the strongest and for the rest of nature. From an eco-system's perspective, death is just as beneficial as life.

But now back to you, our hominid hunter, who has some level of self-awareness. In this same situation you now have a choice. Paradoxically, it is exactly because you are able to separate yourself from the other that you are able to feel for him. You can make assumptions going by how you would feel and how your friend must be feeling now. More importantly, you also have in some miraculous way been freed from the bounds of nature and the bounds of your instinct to make a choice. Can you leave him, knowing that he will be finished off by wild animals? Will you be considering that it is good for the survival of strong genes to leave him and that it will beneficial for the rest of nature? Or will you see nothing but his pain and your pain, but on the other hand the risk to the rest of the group should you all decide to stay with him?

To add to the problem, your mates will now start thinking and feeling along the same lines. Some will argue for leaving him, some will argue for staying with him. You are now experiencing evaluation, judgement and ultimately conflict; conflict within yourself and conflict with others. From our human point of view, we cannot leave an injured mate even at the cost of the rest whom we equally feel for. From nature's point of view we are taking the wrong path as we have deprived it of nutrition at the same time as weakening our genes and therefore threatening our very survival as a species (in the long run).

Duality is becoming apparent as humans decided to move away from their animal compulsions.

Early homo sapiens had split from nature in some way, but not yet completely. He had the ability to override his instinctual choice and make intellectual and emotional choices. He had the ability to judge, and this brought with it conflict. He was self-aware and able to separate his ego from that of others.

At the point that the light bulb went on, homo sapiens left paradise – the place of non-duality, the place of harmony and natural perfection of the cycles of life and death. Being human means being in a state of conflict, being able to choose and being apart from nature.

As we said before, a further attribute of humans is to be able to anticipate the far future and remember the distant past. This ability is our worst enemy but may well turn out to be our only saving grace in the present age.

If you can anticipate and remember you can consciously do things an animal can only do in the framework and timescales of evolution:

1) you can collect conscious experiences,
2) you get anxious because you remember negative incidents and you know they are likely to occur again,
3) you can learn from experience and plan ahead to change your life for the better.

But however beneficial it may seem to us, ultimately, the tendency to dwell on the past and the future is the root of chronic disease. This is because it is this very ability that made us try to change the future and made us embark on the long miasmatic road.

Back to our friend, the early hunter-gatherer. You and the rest of the group survived the night outside the camp, by sheer luck, it seems. The next days go by in a general feeling of relief. Then, slowly it dawns on you – it will happen again, sooner or later. At the next hunt, you feel a little uncomfortable and somehow distracted. Will you be the next one? Will your mates leave you? Luckily, nothing happens and all is safe later on at camp. A few days later, you begin to feel unsettled again. What if wild animals attack and somehow get past the guards? It could happen, it happened not so long ago. A million years previous to this your animal ancestor did not have the capacity to anticipate. It was not in his programme for the survival of the species, because it may have stopped him from attempting seemingly heroic things necessary for the survival of the fittest.

Now, you are able to anticipate and to take action that may be opposing this very law the whole of nature operates by. You may for instance take precautions such as increasing the number and size of fires around the camp to deter wild animals. By doing this you obviously increase the chance of your own survival, but inadvertently enable a physically weaker man to survive as well as a stronger one. On the one hand the human gene pool becomes weaker and on the other hand an animal goes hungry; in this way the consequences of a human's ability to anticipate opposes nature's laws.

We see that being able to anticipate means opening the door to anxiety. And this anxiety may fuel positive change. But however intense at this point in evolution, I believe that anxiety was intermittent, i.e. happening on and off. It was also beneficial in that it stimulated man into action to find a relief, or some way to get out of a difficult situation. I therefore see this intermittent anxiety as a useful and positive addition to the toolbox available to man. It took a much more decisive change for anxiety to become chronic and therefore detrimental.

The Dawn of Spirituality

It is important to understand that nothing much had changed in the outer circumstances – humans were still hunting and gathering, living in small groups and going about their daily survival routine. But what had changed was their perception! Some of them, perhaps all of them, could now feel intermittent anxiety. What before was their natural habitat with all its dangers, perils, riches and pleasures, had not been intellectually questioned, but just accepted. Now an interesting development occurred – our natural habitat became threatening to us. Our perception had changed. Everywhere we looked, danger could be lurking. Experience told us so. We had left paradise. Genesis was right after all.

Thank God for duality, because now one of the most important aspects of our psyche became apparent – out of the need to mentally and emotionally survive the perception of threat, we came up with spirituality. We became aware of, or we invented (you may decide for yourself), a benevolent force that could protect us from danger. This became part of human consciousness to such a degree that it is almost impossible to say whether it is just an invention of a desperate psyche or a necessary building block of the human experience, installed to ensure the survival of the species.

Unfortunately, this saving grace nurtured our next peril – enslaved by fear of angering the benevolent force, we had yet another reason to be anxious. More about this later, but for now let us recognise that this spirituality offered a solution to anxiety.

What has any of this to do with miasms and chronic disease?

Everything, because it perfectly describes the mental/ emotional picture of the susceptibility to Psora. We have not yet arrived at full-blown Psora as some aspects are missing, such as chronic anxiety, despair and the most important link – the disease stimulus. As we will see below, we are actually missing chronic disease itself.

Did Early Humans get Sick?

There is evidence of severe trauma to bones such as skull fractures and vertebral fusions, all due to accidents and injury. There is also evidence of infection. Due to many diseases expressing in soft tissue we cannot say for sure whether early man got chronically ill along the lines of diabetes, cancer or heart disease. We can however make justified assumptions.

Early man was a hunter-gatherer, there is no doubt about it. Present day hunter-gatherer societies such as the !Kung in Botswana are virtually clear of chronic disease such as cancer, heart disease and diabetes, although their DNA is identical to ours.[1] They are Homo sapiens just as much as we are, yet deep chronic disease is almost unknown amongst them. Their life expectancy is similar to ours – 10 per cent of their population are 60 years or older. As a comparison, in 2000, the US had 12.4 per cent of their population at pensionable age of 65 or over.

We also have historical reports of explorers such as this one by Captain Cook, writing about his visit to New Zealand in 1772 "...A further proof that human nature is here

---

1 Lee, R.B. The Kung Bushmen of Botswana. In Hunters and Gatherers Today, M.G. Bicchieri, ed., pp. 327-35. New York: Holt, Rinehart and Winston, 1972.

O'Keefe JH Jr, Cordain L. Cardiovascular disease resulting from a diet and lifestyle at odds with our Paleolithic genome: how to become a 21st century hunter-gatherer. Mayo Clin Proc. 2004; 79 (1), 101-108.

untainted with disease is the great number of old men that we saw... appeared to be very ancient, yet none of them were decrepit; and though not equal in the young in muscular strength, were not a whit behind them in cheerfulness and vivacity." [2]

In 1564 the French explorer Rene de Laudonniere wrote about native Indians in Florida "The agility of the women is so great that they can swim over great rivers, bearing their children upon one of their arms. They climb up, also, very nimbly upon the highest of trees in the country... even the most ancient women of the country dance with the others." [3]

In South America, a tribe of Indians called the Yanomano did not know salt until the early 1970's. They lived a "non-Westernized" lifestyle and their average population blood pressure remained at around 100/65 till old age.[4]

Back to our early humans.

We can probably safely assume that early humans had a very low, if any, incidence of deep (metabolic) chronic disease.

There is however plenty of evidence of acute disease such as trauma to bones and teeth as well as degenerative joint disease and infection. Degenerative joint and tooth disease is evident in Neanderthal remains and it could be that a diet exclusively based on meat would encourage such degeneration due to an acid overload. Too much acidity in

---

2   Cook, J.A. Voyage Towards the South Pole and Round the World. London: W.Strathan & T.Cadell, 1777.

3   Laudonniere, R.G. Histoire Notable de la Florida. Gainsville: University of Florida Press, 1975.

4   Oliver, W.J., Cohen, E.L., and Neel, J.V. Blood pressure, sodium intake, and sodium related hormones in the Yanomano Indians, a 'no-salt' culture. Circulation, 1975 Jul; 52 91: 146-51

our body tissues encourages calcium loss from bones and teeth and this is what may have happened to Neanderthal man. After all, he did disappear and was replaced by Cro-Magnon, a Homo sapiens, who ate meat and plants.

Acute disease such as physical trauma and infection is part of life and can be seen in all living organisms. It is a way of sorting the weak from the strong, a way of encouraging the fittest to pass on their genes. Once you survive acute disease you are fit to continue (unless a physical disability remains as in the case of some bone fractures).

How did this acute picture common to all living organisms shift to the chronic, only seen in humans and domesticated animals?

Susceptibility and Disease Stimulus

Disease comes into being through a marriage of susceptibility and disease stimulus. This was clearly stated by Hahnemann and since then it has been found to be true even by proponents of conventional medicine.

We sometimes forget that it applies to miasms too. It means that each miasm only came into being through the meeting of a particular susceptibility with a matching (similar) disease stimulus. No susceptibility, no miasm. So where did Psora come from?

If the fundamental miasm Psora, i.e. chronic disease as such, was caused by an infection (the stimulus) – as some homeopaths believe – it must have met with an original susceptibility. So far nobody succeeded in clearly defining this susceptibility beyond some very general statements. If we ever want to see ourselves being accepted by mainstream medicine or a critical mass of the general public, we need to be more precise.

In my opinion, the most satisfying written explanation of why humans attracted chronic disease is given by Colin Griffiths in his "Companion to Homeopathy".[5] Griffiths seems to believe that susceptibility to Psora came out of a general state of dread, hunger, anticipation, anxiety and restlessness afflicting humans since they acquired awareness. He does not go much further into this, but hints at a story similar to the one told more expansively by myself above. For Griffiths the susceptibility or weakness that predisposed us to chronic disease was mostly in the mental /emotional sphere, although his mentioning "hunger" seems to indicate physical issues too. He then continues that this susceptibility was met with scabies, a parasitic infection that affected only those who were weakened. The difference between the effect of scabies and that of other acute infection is, in Griffith's view, a combination of factors to do with the location of the infection and the evolutionary success of parasites in general. This is why scabies became incurable and miasmatic and other acute infections did not.

Although this line of thought seems close to being satisfactory, it is not completely so (although I may of course have missed something or misunderstood any aspect of Griffith's explanation). The following remains to be answered.

Why did scabies and not any other parasite bring us to our knees?

5   Watkins, London 2005.

If the susceptibility was all mental/emotional, was this imbalance really strong enough to cause a change so significant that a parasite such as the scabies mites could not be overcome by our otherwise so invincible life force?

Why, until quite recently, were there societies untouched by chronic disease? Did they never acquire anxiety to those levels that would cause chronic disease and if not, why not?

Why would our species that had evolved according to the laws of natural evolution, perfect in every aspect for the ecological niche it inhabited, be anxious to such a degree that it became so extremely vulnerable? Anxiety must have a function in the eyes of evolution, but only a life-preserving one, never an annihilating one! Surely human beings developed so-called negative emotions as tools, red flags or warning signals, so they could react and adapt to avoid danger.

So why did we acquire this weakness that left us defenceless against scabies?

As we will see, the heart of the matter lies in the just-mentioned ecological niche. In fact, Griffith's "hunger", his only representation of a physical susceptibility to Psora, can be more adequately expanded into a web of interplaying physical factors deriving from a change to the ecological niche homo sapiens chose to inhabit from a particular time onwards. In effect, homo sapiens fell victim to Psora because he left the niche he had perfectly evolved for. Just as our pets fall victims to cancer because they are not living according to their evolutionary design (canned food, no exercise, environmental pollution, vaccines, etc), we began deteriorating because we left "paradise", our original birthplace.[6]

Although this may come as a surprise to the reader, the following pages will explain why I believe this to be true.

The Law of Similars

To begin with, the key to understanding chronic disease is found by looking not very far, but nearby at our own laws. The law of similars for instance.

We know that disease energy and disease susceptibility must be similar, i.e. of similar quality and quantity. This similarity in quality can be translated into a logical match such as the match of fear of loneliness (susceptibility) matched with an actual abandonment (stimulus). A fear of loneliness would not be matched by something completely unrelated such as a dog bite. If the match is logically related, then disease will ensue. In our example of loneliness and abandonment we would perhaps see a Pulsatilla pathology emerging. In the other, logically not related example there is no match and so no chronic pathology will emerge.

The similarity in quantity of susceptibility and stimulus refers to the strength, severity or depth of the events. A matching example would be the depth of fear of sudden death and a severe non-fatal car crash bringing about a

---

6   O'Keefe JH Jr, Cordain L. Cardiovascular disease resulting from a diet and lifestyle at odds with our Paleolithic genome: how to become a 21st century hunter-gatherer. Mayo Clin Proc 2004 Jan; 79(1):101-8.

Kowalski LM, Bujko J. Evaluation of biological and clinical potential of paleolithic diet. Rocz Panstw Zakl Hig. 2012; 63(1):9-15.

Jönsson T, Ahrén B, et al. A Paleolithic diet confers higher insulin sensitivity, lower C-reactive protein and lower blood pressure than a cereal-based diet in domestic pigs. Nutr Metab (Lond). 2006 Nov 2; 3:39.

Frassetto LA, Schloetter M et al. Metabolic and physiologic improvements from consuming a paleolithic, hunter-gatherer type diet. Eur J Clin Nutr. 2009 Aug; 63(8):947-55

heart attack in a surviving driver. But if the fear of sudden death meets with burning your hand lightly on the iron, no chronic pathology will ensue. This is because the depth of fear would in most cases not be matched by the trivial problem of a light burn.

Transferring this understanding to Psora, we must identify a susceptibility that is a true similar match with the stimulus. If we believe that scabies was the stimulus, we must find a susceptibility that is similar in quality and quantity, i.e. logically related and of similar severity or depth.

Before I go further into this, first let us try to demystify and express in ordinary language the concept of susceptibility and stimulus.

If we think it through carefully, we can see that we only get chronically sick if a particular attitude or mental/emotional state causes specific, health damaging behaviours (possibly in the previous generation). It may be the behaviour itself or a secondary behaviour or associated environmental factor which causes damage. But it is never the original attitude itself, alone, that makes us sick.

For example, the attitude of boredom (susceptibility) is likely to cause depression or perhaps aggression. Depression may cause alcohol abuse (a damaging behaviour). This in turn causes chronic disease such as liver or bowel disease. In others, depression may cause lack of energy and poor motivation. A depressed person may therefore engage in little else than sleeping and, being unable to earn his own living, he thereby opens the door to health problems due to poor diet and lifestyle choices. You can see that boredom (or depression) itself does not make anyone sick but, combined with the compensating behaviour, it does.

In the case of cancer, a susceptibility exists (commonly accepted in scientific circles as a presence of latent cancer genes), but the disease only comes to expression if certain environmental factors stimulate it into existence, or as some call it "switch on the gene". It is our attitude which allows these environmental factors to exist (pollution, toxicity, electro-smog etc) and, for our purpose, carcinogenic environmental factors are therefore classed as a consequence of our planet-polluting behaviours. Cancer is therefore only possible if and when toxins or pollution hit a cancer gene. And since most of us have cancer genes and most of us are subject to a critical mass of toxic pollution, we are all at risk. But more about this later.

In addition, I believe that the disease stimulus is hardly ever a single factor, but usually multi-factorial. This view should not be intimidating or discouraging, but empowering. It enables us to address disease from various angles and allows us to take responsibility in many ways.

Attitude, Behaviour and Chronic Disease

Susceptibility is a specific attitude, such as "ailments from business failure" being an Aurum attitude/susceptibility.[7] The person remains stuck in the attitude because the organism somehow perceives this attitude to be advantageous, i.e. better than the previous alternative they were stuck in.

---

7   An Aurum person afflicted in this way will not try again in business, as their present pain is so great that they simply will not want to repeat the experience. This attitude is seen as advantageous as it prevents a repetition of a painful experience, but it does nothing to remove the ailment as the Aurum–type personalities stay stuck in their perception that business failure causes them pain. As long as they have the attitude, they will have the pain and continue the tendency to feel pain from failures in the future.

Let us remember that the vital force is always self-preserving. This is key – any altered susceptibility/attitude must be advantageous. Any alternative would be worse.

Further, for susceptibility to predispose to miasmatic (chronic) disease, the susceptibility – or attitude – must also be chronic (miasmatic) to some degree. There has to be a similar match. By this I mean that the attitude could not be easily altered and that the human species as a whole or large population groups must have been stuck in it with no way out. If there had been many different attitudes/susceptibilities we would have had a choice and would not all have moved in the same direction. But we did all acquire Psora and therefore must have made the same choice. It follows that we must have all had an identical attitude/susceptibility. And only the most advantageous attitude would have prevailed. Therefore we all, collectively, must have been stuck in something we perceived to be advantageous. Only then would our behaviour have changed dramatically and for very long periods – enough to be able to cause a trans-generational layer of chronic disease.

If this had not been so, how could a universal miasmatic picture have emerged and collectively changed the human experience from a usually healthy life with short, intense disease incidents to a life tainted by low-level, constant or recurring health complaints?

> The attitude must have changed collectively without any alternative being available, or it must have been the most advantageous attitude.
> The attitude must have changed in a most dramatic way.

> The attitude must have changed and remained changed for many generations.

> A matching disease stimulus/behaviour must have met this attitude in order for physical disease or Psoric symptoms to emerge.

> This behaviour must also have been dramatic and be present for many generations to continuously re-establish and reinforce the Psoric picture until it was impossible for a critical mass to recover by evolutionary pathways or newly-found solutions.

Psora

Back to our pre-Psoric hunter gatherer in Africa, Europe and Asia. He is showing mental/emotional signs and attitudes of Psora, but he is not chronically sick yet.

Some may think it was just a matter of time before man got sick once he gained consciousness. Maybe so. Maybe intermittent anxiety as described above was enough to weaken his immunes system in a way that it could not throw off our Hahnemannian disease stimulus[8] – a parasitic infection causing scabies.

But this is not quite logical. In fact, if you believe this reasoning, then any parasitic infection could have taken hold at this point. Many wild animals carry parasites and live with them. I suspect that humans were hosts to the scabies mite as well as other parasites (including bowel parasites) for a long time but never had much of a problem with them. One wonders why a more or less harmless infestation with parasites transformed into bothersome symptoms that could not ever be healed? Symptoms which were

---

8   It is not clear whether Hahnemann thought of Psora as caused by infection. He used the German term "Krätze", but this term can and could be used generally for red itchy skin without referring to scabies as such.

transmitted to the next generation if suppressed? Perhaps this happened at a point when our intermittent anxiety reached levels that reduced our immune defence enough to tip the scales in favour of parasites, enabling them to take over. Or perhaps other factors were responsible for weakening our system to the degree where parasites could take a hold beyond the harmless. In any case it seems illogical to assume that only one type of parasite was present; it must have been several different ones.

Parasites

Let's look at parasites more closely. As I mentioned before, any animal (including humans) is host to parasites at any time. But parasites can only produce bothersome symptoms if our system is weakened by other factors. For instance, some bowel parasites need an alkaline bowel environment to flourish. Skin parasites and fungi also need a change of skin pH to alkaline in order to produce symptoms.[9] It may therefore be that parasitic infections producing Psoric symptoms were accompanied by a change in the environment of the host's body. How would such a change come about? We know that our emotions can change our internal biochemical environment; in this way intermittent anxiety would have played a part. But we also know that other basic prerequisites for health such as diet, sleep, exercise etc all have an influence on our immune system and general body biochemical environment. If there had been a negative change in Psoric man with respect to all or some of these factors, severe parasitic infection on an epidemic scale would be likely. If the only problem for man was occasional

---

9   Yosipovitch G, Hu J. The Importance of Skin pH: Skin & aging. 2003; 11(3): 88-93.

anxiety, I do not believe his immune system would have been sufficiently weakened to attract a horrendous disease such as scabies or leprosy. There is no energetic match.

This is the reason why I do not believe that scabies caused Psora.

We know that disease stimulus and susceptibility have to be logically related and be equal in their energy. In other words, they have to match just like symptoms need to match remedy. But I believe that scabies was too severe and early hunter-gatherer man was too healthy to catch it! There was no match. (He did of course live with parasites, but these did not bother him too much.)

In the case of scabies we know that it can literally drive an infected person crazy. The itch is intolerable and people will tear themselves to shreds scratching their skin. This must surely be one of the most horrendous experiences, and not much relief was available for early man. It is also highly contagious and so nobody was safe. Infected people were most likely isolated from the group. This in itself as well as the intolerable itch must have been an absolutely terrifying perspective for early man. In leprosy the story is similar.

I believe that man's intermittent anxiety caused by survival issues was no match for the kind of terrifying energy that scabies as stimulus presented man with. I believe that the anxiety was not strong enough. Man was too healthy to get scabies at this stage. He was still living in his usual environment, the one he had perfectly evolved for. He had all the tools – physical, emotional and mental – available to him to preserve the species, in the same way as any other perfectly evolved wild animal did. The only difference to a wild animal was the awareness that he had acquired; an awareness which brought with it a new set of tools (anxiety, anticipation, judgement etc) that were felt intermittently but employed positively to preserve life. These tools would not have evolved otherwise. This is a very important point in our discussion – the newly evolved emotions that Griffiths quotes as susceptibilities to disease, were in my eyes positive additions to our toolbox. They would not have made us ill by themselves, because they were not overpoweringly strong enough nor permanent enough to overwhelm our vital force in such a life-changing way that a miasm would afford. According to my view, man still lived in his original habitat in all respects and he was in no way weakened to such a degree as to be susceptible to a horrendous disease such as scabies.

Therefore I suggest that Psora was not caused by any infection, but that infectious skin diseases were a result of Psora! Whoever started the rumour of scabies causing Psora did not go back far enough because he did not have the information that we have now. More about this later.

The realisation that scabies was a result of Psora will logically ask for another, gentler disease stimulus to meet and marry with early man's intermittent survival anxiety as susceptibility. Once the marriage was consummated, man's health began to decline sufficiently for scabies to take hold.

There is really no way around it but to accept that chronic disease existed before scabies. Sankaran in his "Schema"[10] expressed a similar view by placing 2-3 miasms before Psora, or indeed as collectively replacing Psora. For me, all of these first disease states are just a natural progression of mild to severe Psora as we will see that they all have the

10 Homeopathic Medical Publishers, Mumbai, 2005

same susceptibility/mental attitude as well as the same stimulus/behaviour at their root.

For homeopaths today this insight has important consequences. All our anti-miasmatic remedies are chosen for their ability to reduce the miasmatic influences as defined by the diseases we have assumed to be their cause. But if the disease did not cause the miasm, our time-line of chronic disease looks very different. And our treatment of chronic disease should too.

Using Psorinum and anti-Psoric remedies will only get us back to the state of health before scabies came on the scene. It will only cure some of the Psoric picture, i.e. that part which is related to the scabies stimulus. This is because we have defined anti-Psoric to be anti-scabies (or "anti-a-similar-state-to-scabies"). But this state of health is not perfect health. It is still Psoric. Psoric; with all its digestive, liver, kidney lung and skin symptoms and with all its anxiety and depression. We are just moving from deeper Psora to milder Psora and this is probably what we mean when we say that we can only put miasm to sleep, not completely eradicate it. We need to know more about Psora before scabies made an impact.[11]

So what was the matching disease stimulus that initially moved early man into the chronic picture of (mild) Psora? What happened before scabies? And is this what we are missing in the puzzle of chronic disease?

---

11 Even if you do not buy into the concept of Psora being caused by scabies, but prefer a concept based more on disease energy, you still have to accept that you are trying to cure your idea of Psora with remedies based on other people's incorrect assumptions.

The Agricultural Revolution

30,000 – 10,000 years ago man opted out of the food chain he had been a part of so far. He left the ecological niche he had inhabited and stopped being prey and hunting prey (in both cases not exclusively but for the most part). Man settled down, began planting grass seeds on a large scale and thus solved his most basic survival issues – food and shelter. Fossil records of the earliest crude stone grinding tools date back to 13,000 years ago, which means that by that time cereals were definitely on the menu.[12] Man also began domesticating animals, but we will discuss this later.

Planting our food freed us of time spent hunting and gathering and it supplied a surplus of calories. In spite of this surplus, most people needed to work harder than before, because agriculture is a time consuming business.[13] Luckily, some very few people managed to spend less time doing physical work and could concentrate on more mental activities. In time, advanced tools could be invented and animals were domesticated to relieve humans to some degree of hard manual labour.

Life became safer as settlements grew and became non-natural oases in the middle of nature. This alone kept wild animals at bay as these settlements were not something animals could recognise as hunting ground. In addition, some small scale division of labour and exchange of goods against labour must have started at this stage. Some people began tentatively exploring more academic pursuits, with their spare energy being diverted to their mind. They began

12 Wright, K. The origins and development of ground stone assemblages in Late Pleistocene South-West Asia. Paleorient, 1991; 17:19-45

13 Gladwell M. The Outliers - the story of success. 2008. London: Allen Lane

pondering mathematical and astronomical questions as well as putting effort into first writing and reading.

On the whole then, man was better off. The situation was advantageous and nobody really wanted to go back.

First, food was available all year round, as man had learnt how to store cereals in granaries. Second, cereals provided a large proportion of the daily caloric needs, and hunting and gathering could be reduced dramatically or stopped altogether. (Man also began cultivating vegetables and fruit). Less hunting, fewer accidents and injuries, less intense pain and less death. Less upset and upheaval.

Life was good, or at least better than before. But was it healthier?

In fact, the seed of chronic disease that was planted when we left paradise was now able to germinate in the Pre-Psoric soil of intermittent anxiety. Recently, evidence has appeared showing a dramatic increase in chronic disease, mal-nutrition and even a reduction in life-expectancy from the moment man began growing his own food.[14] (Interestingly, an increase in acute infectious disease was also noted.) But why now? Why did full-blown Psora (not just the mental-emotional picture but the physical expression) emerge now?

Why exactly man turned to agriculture is not known, but one plausible theory is that in the millennia before the first

---

14 Cohen MN and Armelagos GJ, eds. Paleopathology at the Origin of Agriculture. New York: Academic Press. 1994

Steckel RH and Jerome C. The Backbone of History: Health and Nutrition in the Western Hemisphere. Cambridge: 2002; Cambridge University Press

Robson AJ. A Bioeconomic View of the Neolithic Transition to Agriculture. Canadian Journal of Economics. 2010; 43(1):280-300

agricultural revolution, food supply was becoming sparse.[15] This may have been because of population expansion or because of other events that led to a decline in prey. Therefore the survival of the species was under threat. Remember that we were hunting and gathering. Too many clans on the turf would graze off each other's berries and disturb the prey. From a homeopath's point of view, scarcity of food is of course a majorly Psoric issue.

Man had at this point been intermittently anxious about basic survival issues (food and shelter) for many millennia. He had solved some of his problems by inventing, or becoming aware of, a benevolent force who could protect him. However, at some point intelligent man realised that disaster could strike in any case, regardless of all the sacrifices and rites he performed to appease his god(s). On the one hand this increased anxiety levels for many individuals. On the other hand some less anxious but rather more frustrated individuals fuelled the next, most significant step for mankind. To not be completely at the mercy of these rather moody gods, and to solve his increasing problem of food supply, intelligent man decided to grow his own food.

This process must have taken place over centuries if not millennia (due to the necessary gathering of knowledge and experience and of course time needed for cultivation of wild plants into agriculturally valuable crops), but scientific evidence tells us that growing crops became fashionable about 10,000 years ago.

---

15 Cohen MN. The Food Crisis in Prehistory: Overpopulation and The Originsof Agriculture. New Haven. 1977; Yale University Press

Cereals

The agricultural revolution took place in north-east Africa and in near-by Middle East. Some animal husbandry also became popular, but to the significantly greater part, man became reliant on grains to cover his ever-expanding appetite. This was a major change in diet. Probably up to 70% of calories was now supplied by grains. These had never been on the menu before except perhaps in minute amounts that could be secured by gathering. Prior to cultivation, grains were just grasses. How much nutrition can you get out of some grass seeds? Would it be worthwhile collecting these if a banana tree was growing next door?

Cereals, such as wheat, rye, barley, oats and rice, can be digested by humans as long as they are cooked. The nutrition we get out of them is glucose. The starches in cereals are converted into sugars and ultimately to glucose. This is the fuel we (mostly) run on.

What most people do not realise is that along with glucose, cereals also provide us with a lot of grief.

Acidity

To start with, all cereals leave acidity in our tissues when we actually require alkalinity.[16] Meat, dairy and pulses also do this. The problem is that cereals are eaten in far larger quantities than these other items just mentioned. And this means that we do not have enough room left to eat enough alkaline-forming foods to balance the acidity. Cereals crowd

---

16 Remer, T. Infuence of nutrition on acid-base balance – metabolic aspects. European Jouranl of Nutrition, 2001; 40:214-20.

Remer T, Manz F. Potential renal acid load of foods and its influence on urine pH. Journal of the American Dietetic Association.1995; 95:791-97

Sebastian A, Frassetto LA. et al.Estimation of the net acid load of the diet of ancestral preagricultural Homo sapiens and their hominid ancestors. American Journal of Clinical Nutrition. 2002; 76:1,308-16

alkaline-forming foods out of our diet. Look at your break-fast, lunch and dinner plate. How much of it is covered in cereals? Often it is than half if not three quarters of it! This means that your soft tissues and especially your connective tissues will become acidic when ideally they need to be alkaline. In turn, your body reacts by withdrawing alkaline minerals from your teeth and bones to attempt to get back to normal. This is because every one of your cells needs an alkaline medium in which to conduct chemical reactions. But the human body is resilient. It will tolerate many years of increasing acidity before showing signs of distress. This is why, in our minds and awareness, we never linked cereals to health problems.

Minerals and Vitamin B

So what else is wrong with cereals (even wholegrains)?

Eating cereals produces vitamin and mineral deficiency. This is due to several factors. To start with, calorie for calorie, cereals are poor in minerals and vitamins compared to vegetables, fruit and animal flesh.

In addition, Zinc, Copper, Calcium and Iron levels become reduced due to the phytate content in cereals (and pulses!). Phytates will bind to those minerals and carry them out in your stool. This is one reason why vegetarians are more at risk from becoming anaemic. (The other reason is that vegetarian iron is less well absorbed.)

Vitamins most at risk are the vitamin B group, as cereals contain much less vitamin B compared to vegetables and animal flesh. Interestingly, the vitamin B group and Magnesium are intimately involved in energy release from glucose. Eating cereals will therefore make you tired.

Cereals are also low in vitamin A/beta-carotene and they contain no vitamin C. Of course one could make up the deficit by eating a lot of fruit and vegetables, but unfortunately most of us fill up on cereals to such an extent that there is simply not enough room left for the amounts of fruit and vegetables required to make up this deficit.

Where will this lead to after several years of covering your dinner plate and snack pack with cereals? It will lead to a deficiency of vitamins and minerals, even though you are eating every day until your stomach is full. You will not notice at first, but you will after several years (but again you will not link your health problems to what you are eating). Particular minerals at risk are Magnesium, Zinc, Chromium, Iron and Copper.

What is more, a woman deficient to some mild degree, will pass on this deficiency to her offspring, especially during repeated pregnancies. The fifth child will be in worse health than the first, because the mother is never able to make good her deficiencies and becomes more and more depleted as she keeps reproducing. After all, pregnancy is one of the most physiologically and nutritionally demanding processes of the human body.

Here we have our first hint of how a problem can become miasmatic. And we managed to explain this in very simple and conventional terms.

Lectins

Grains, especially wheat, but also many types of beans and pulses (as well as dairy) are high in proteins called lectins. Lectins routinely attach to parts of our gut wall, making it more porous by way of inducing inflammation.[17] The damage is not confined to the digestive tract, however. Lectins have been found to be associated with systemic immune and endocrine problems.[18] One particular substance called wheat germ agglutinin (WGA), is especially vicious and can bring about immune, endocrine, cytotoxic, cardiovascular and neurological dysfunction.[19] There is also some evidence of gliadin, another protein found in wheat, barley, rye and oats causing increased intestinal permeability regardless of genetic susceptibility to coeliac disease.[20]

In atopic individuals (i.e. people with eczema, asthma or hay fever) some lectins can trigger the release of IgE antibodies, inducing a classic allergic reaction detectable by medical skin-prick tests.[21]

17 Guzyeyeva GV. Lectin glycosylation as a marker of thin gut inflammation. The Faseb Journal. 2008; 22:898.3

18 Pusztai A. Dietary lectins are metabolic signals for the gut and modulate immune and hormone functions. Eur J Clin Nutr. 1993 Oct; 47(10):691-9.

19 Dalla Pellegrina C, et al. Effects of wheat germ agglutinin on human gastrointestinal epithelium: insights from an experimental model of immune/epithelial cell interaction. Toxicol Appl Pharmacol. 2009 Jun 1; 237(2):146-53. Epub 2009 Mar 28

    Pusztai A, Ewen SW, et al. Antinutritive effects of wheat-germ agglutinin and other N-acetylglucosamine-specific lectins.Br J Nutr. 1993 Jul; 70(1):313-21

    Tchernychev B, Wilchek M. Natural human antibodies to dietary lectins. FEBS Lett. 1996 Nov 18; 397(2-3):139-42

    Liu WK, Sze SC, Ho JC, Liu BP, Yu MC. Wheat germ lectin induces G2/M arrest in mouse L929 fibroblasts. J Cell Biochem. 2004 Apr 15; 91(6):1159-73.

    Ohmori T, Yatomi Y. et al. Wheat germ agglutinin-induced platelet activation via platelet endothelial cell adhesion molecule-1: involvement of rapid phospholipase C gamma 2 activation by Src family kinases. Biochemistry. 2001 Oct 30; 40(43):12992-3001

20 Drago S, et al. Gliadin, zonulin and gut permeability: effects on celiac and non-celiac intestinal mucosa and intestinal cell lines. Scand J Gastroenterol. 2006; 41(4):408-19.

    Assimakopoulos SF et al. Enterocytes' tight junctions: From molecules to diseases. World J Gastrointest Pathophysiol, 2011; 15;2(6):123-37.

21 Cordain, L., Toohey L. etal. Modulation of Immune Function by Dietary Lectins in Rheumatoid Arthritis. Br J Nutr 2000; 83:207-217

Mould

Once cereals are processed, i.e. milled and baked, they are prone to mould infestation. In fact, nowadays most bakery goods contain calcium propionate, or E282, which is supposed to stop mould from growing. (This preservative comes with its own problems.) Early settler would not have had any preservative available to stop mould from forming in his bread, although eating bread straight after baking would have prevented much of this problem. It really only became prominent later on, when Sycosis emerged. But even now it added to the load of unfavourable factors associated with the new diet of early settler. Mould is toxic in our system and weakens our immune system. This makes us prone to other infections taking hold.[22]

Slowing Down

Looking at what acidity and mineral/vitamin deficiency alone can do in our body, we must conclude that the very first effect is a general slowing down of normal chemical processes in all body cells. For instance, a lack of magnesium has an effect on cell membrane pumps. There are different types of these and they help to move substances in and out of all cells. If less can get in and less can get out, a cell will lack important ingredients and will get filled up with waste. This will bring a slowing down of cellular processes. A slowing down; an underfunction. Psora.

Not convinced? There is more.

---

22 Gray MR, Thrasher JD et al. Mixed mould mycotoxicosis: immunological changes in humans following exposure in water-damaged buildings. Arch Envirn Health. 2003 Jul; 58(7):410-20

Addiction

Cereals have an opiate effect.[23] Eating cereals causes a temporary change in our brain chemistry. In other words, they make us feel good for a while, beyond the normal satisfaction we get out of not feeling hungry. This effect lasts a few hours and then turns into the opposite. We feel lousy. Not only because we are hungry, but because we have come down from the drugging effect. In fact cereals are a downer for most people; they calm us down and help us sleep. What happens to us now would have happened to the first settlers too. They are the same homo sapiens that we are now. We have not changed in our body chemistry at all. No truly genetic adaptation (change in the structure of our DNA) has taken place. In fact the only adaptation that has taken place is the shift from acute Psoric upsets that were more common in the past to more chronic Psoric upsets that are more common now.

Back to our settlers – they ate their bread, were calm and happy for a while and then suddenly got all nervy and anxious again. What did they do? What do you do? You have more of the same because you associate the good feeling with a particular behaviour. In time we need more to get the same effect. This is called conditioning and we all know it. We just don't want to admit it when it comes to cereals. Why? Because we are addicted and this clouds our awareness. We cannot see beyond our personal awareness. We cannot see where we went wrong.

23 Kitts DD, Weiler K. Bioactive proteins and peptides from food sources. Applications of bioprocesses used in isolation and recovery. Curr Pharm Des. 2003; 9(16):1309-23

Teschemacher H. Opioid receptor ligands derived from food proteins. Curr Pharm Des. 2003; 9(16):1331-44.

Sioudrou et al. Opioid peptides derived from food proteins. The exorphins. J Biol Chem.1979; 254:2446-2449.

Admittedly, cereals cause a much milder addiction than, for instance, cocaine. But it is still an addiction. Addiction strains our chemical balance as we are going from an unnatural low to an unnatural high. Our body must expend extra resources to rebalance itself from such unnatural states. I repeat, it was a mild addiction that early man suffered from, but it made a start and certainly contributed to the emergence of chronic disease.

Cereals and Anxiety

Interestingly, there was another reason why cereals became so popular. I just mentioned it in the previous paragraph – cereals calm us down. Cereals fell on the fertile soil of the anxious Psoric mind and helped him to calm his nerves. The problem is that when the calming effect wore off, anxiety returned and he needed to reach for more.

But why was man still anxious now? Had he not solved his basic survival issues of food and shelter?

Chronic Background Anxiety

The truth is that early settler man had only exchanged a very acute but intermittent anxiety with a more chronic one as you will see below. On top of this he had one more thing to worry about now – new types of diseases emerged that were harder to get rid of or that never properly resolved. How come?

Imagine you are living in an early settlement somewhere in Mesopotamia. This year the harvest was not so good. There was a drought and not much grew. You have not been able to fill the granaries. You are worried that till the next planting season you may have to resort to hunting and fishing. But the rivers are running low and large game and fish are scarce in and around the rivers. You are also worried about the little grain you have been able to store. Would pests be bad this year? How many mice and rats will there be and what about that strange mould that attacked your stores last season? You would have to eat the grain anyway, even if it looked bad. You had no choice.

Thus the more acute and intermittent anxiety about the threatening world around early hunter gatherer was exchanged for a lower intensity chronic anxiety about the weather, the harvest, and pests attacking the food stores.[24]

Disease Agents

On another note, your cesspit behind one of the huts has to be cleared out. You have noticed many flies and other insects around that area and you were wondering whether they might have a go at your grain stores too. In fact you are not aware of the much bigger threat to your well-being these little pests pose – after feeding on your faeces they will settle on your food which is now only several meters away from where you dropped your stool (festering away with the other people's and attracting a thriving population of germ transmitting insects and parasites). Before settlements were common, people used to discreetly disappear behind some bush or tree and perhaps cover whatever they left behind with leaves. Only the odd fly would find their way from there to your food, there was simply too much distance between. In settlements, there would have been a

---

24 Tutankhamun's Cat: Why do two main Psoric remedies (Sulph and Calc) adore cats (and not dogs)? Because cats catch mice. And mice eat grain. Psoric man relied on grain for his survival! So cats became his best friend. Perhaps for this reason, ancient Egyptians elevated cats to god status.

Nowadays many people believe that cats are telepathic and have special healing properties. This is of course a Sycotic type of attitude (clairvoyant), covering up Psoric survival anxiety.

Isn't homeopathy wonderful.

common lavatory where everyone would drop their excrement, probably just behind someone's hut.

Parasites and germs were always part of life even for hunter gatherers, but now their populations were increasing and opportunities to stimulate disease were amass in the more crowded living conditions of early settler. Living conditions produced a critical mass of germs and parasites that not even the healthiest immune system could defend against.

What about your hut? Ventilation is restricted. Your large agricultural family (many children needed to serve the fields) crowds in every night. Fleas, mites and other creepy crawlies which enjoy poorly ventilated, hot and sweaty places will have a field day (or night). Many invisible creatures will feast too (parasites, bacteria).

We can see that by way of settling down and changing our ecological niche, several disease stimuli emerged: an acid-producing diet lower in nutrients and causing an addictive cycle; poor hygiene; higher exposure to disease transmitting or producing germs/parasites.

Yet this is still not the complete story. One very important link is still missing...

Exercise

Hunter gatherers took aerobic exercise many hours per day. Hunting parties spent probably about 2 hrs per day in pursuit of game, often at jogging and running pace. Gathering parties would go at walking speed engaging in light anaerobic activities such as bending, climbing and moving their bodies in all sorts of ways. Hunting and gathering was rotated and alternated so that strength of various muscle groups involved could be recovered.[25]

Once man settled down, the days of chasing game were over. Exercise slowed down and became predominantly anaerobic. The exercise schedule was therefore dramatically altered to zero aerobic activity combined with daily strenuous anaerobic activity of field work. This involved not only the increased use of muscle for strength but also a stronger emphasis on muscle groups of the upper body that were never used to this degree before. In addition, there were no rest days! Anaerobic exercise was engaged in every day and this changed the dietary need for glucose dramatically. Without recovery days, muscle tissue is in great need for quick fuel and this can only be provided if no complicated metabolic conversion from proteins or fats has to take place before it can be used. Farmers were of course in the lucky position to grow exactly the right fuel for their lifestyle – cereals. These are converted into glucose very readily and muscle tissue can be refuelled within minutes after eating. The problem was and still is that cereal consumption brings with it many downsides, as we have seen. After some time on this new regimen, early settler began to use domesticated animals to do most of his heavy work. But he continued eating a large amount of cereals without needing to, and so sped up the chronic disease process by a subtle degree.

Early settler was now caught in a difficult situation – he settled down to grow cereals and he needed to eat cereals in order to be able to grow cereals. Eating vegetables, fruit

25   Cordain L, Gotshall RW, Eaton SB. Evolutionary aspects of exercise. World review of nutrition and diet, 1997; 81:49-60
     Cordain L, Gotshall RW, Eaton SB. Physical activity, energy expenditure and fitness: an evolutionary perspective. Intl J Sports Med. 1998; 19:328-35

and proteins would not have provided him with enough quick-release glucose to engage in field work.

The change to zero aerobic exercise is also significant in another way. Regular aerobic exercise prevents depression and anxiety. The more the heart rate is raised and the longer it remains raised during exercise the more endorphins are released. These make us feel happy and balance our mood. Early man had no choice but to exercise aerobically regularly and so his system was flooded with "happiness chemicals" all the time. Most people who exercise regularly will tell you that a decent aerobic session will keep them satisfied for about 36 hrs. After this they crave more. This type of addiction is not the same as indulging in an exogenous chemical that is damaging to our body chemistry. Endorphins are endogenous and they have a positive effect on our mood. They do not cause a mineral deficiency and they do not strain our homeostatic mechanisms.

Aerobic exercise is beneficial in other ways – it lowers our heart rate during rest (therefore reduces anxiety by this pathway too) and it lowers our blood fats. It also helps to keep our blood sugar even and it regulates our appetite.

Exercise maintains cardiovascular health partially due to the fact that it initiates a release of nitric oxide in our arteries.[26] Nitric oxide prevents the collapse of blood vessels and is instrumental in maintaining cardiovascular health. When exercise levels and nitric oxide levels reduce, the risk of stroke, haemorrhage, arterial spasm, high blood pressure and high cholesterol increase manifold. Interestingly, sufficient levels of nitric oxide can only be produced

---

26 Gielen S, Sandri M, Erbs S, Adams V. Exercise-induced Modulation of Endothelial Nitric Oxide Production. Curr Pharm Biotechnol. http://www.ncbi.nlm.nih.gov/pubmed/21235458 (2011; as at 24th Jan 2012)

when enough protein (especially the amino acid arginine) is consumed.

Both types of exercise raise our metabolic rate, i.e. the rate at which calories are burned and the rate at which all of our cells function. As we exercise, all body cells become more sensitive to thyroid hormones. This means that our body chemical reactions speed up and more calories are burnt.[27] Exercise also increases sensitivity of body cells to insulin[28], which means that our blood sugar balance mechanism becomes more efficient. This benefit became more evidently lacking in later miasms as we will see.

Reducing exercise levels will therefore produce a subtle slowdown of body chemistry. What does this remind you of? Psora, of course. The fact that a lot of anaerobic exercise was engaged in helped reverse this trend to some extent, but it necessitated a high intake of cereals. As we said, our increased need for glucose could not have been covered in any other way. Unfortunately, this change in diet brought with it considerable disadvantages as explained above.

We can see that early settler definitely cut out the benefits of aerobic exercise, although of course still benefitted from anaerobic exercise. He was still more active than many of us are today. But as a general tendency we can observe that a relative lack of endorphins, a relative lack of the other chemical benefits, plus an excess of cereals in the diet would have left early settler in a slightly more vulnerable position.[29]

27 Musnick D. Clinical Approaches to Structural Imbalances in Functional medicine, ch 29, p 481ff

28 Hughes VA, Fiatarone MA et al. Exercise increases muscle GLUT 4 levels and insulin action in subjects with impaired glucose tolerance. Am J Physiol. 264: E855-E862, 1993.

29 Melzer K,Kayser B, Pichard C. Physical activity: the health benefits outweigh the risks. Curr Opin Clin Nutri Metab Care 2004; 7 (6):641-47

The Shift from Acute to Chronic

Let's take stock of the story so far:

Early settler was still anxious. He was concerned with survival on a less intense but more continuous long term level.

Early settler ate a diet that was acid producing and caused a vitamin and mineral deficit which slowed down his body chemistry. This diet also supplied immune system weakening moulds.

Early settler took less aerobic exercise and therefore was now susceptible to depression as well as anxiety. His body statistics (heart rate, blood sugar balance, blood fats) were also not as favourable. His metabolism had slowed down to some extent.

Early settler lived in mildly unhygienic and crowded conditions and was exposed to a critical mass of germs and parasites.

Early settler achieved compensation for the reduction of natural highs (endorphins) and chronic worries with the opiate effect of cereals and alcohol. This strained his homeostatic mechanisms and added to nutrient deficiencies.

But with the help of cereals and alcohol early settler could carry on. And carry on he did, day after day, month after month, year after year. With the same worries, the same hopes and the same disasters that sooner or later caught up with him. Locusts, droughts, epidemics. Unrelenting heat.

Early settler had no choice. He could not go back. That was not an option. It was still better to have a drought every 5 years than to be eaten by a lion tomorrow.

Early settler had developed full blown Psora.

Compared to hunter gatherer, all his cells were slowing down in their activity. His brain chemistry was slowing down too. He became more sedentary and less intensely ready for action. He developed the potential for depression. Sometimes he felt intense despair at his predicament. Drudgery day in day out, heat, dust, slow but strenuous work. But at least he had a roof over his head and a large family who would take care of him as he was getting older. And food growing on his doorstep.

Physical Psora

Under the strain of mental, emotional and physical changes, early settler would have been prone to develop certain conditions. In fact these conditions would have appeared in a fixed order. This order has long been recognised by naturopaths, and as homeopaths we see elements of it represented in our Law of Cure as stipulated by Hering.[30] The Law of Cure implies that there is a certain order in which the body's tissues heal once subjected to homeopathic treatment. It is further implied that this order is not due to homeopathic treatment, but due to an innate organisational hierarchy of the human body. This always aims to preserve the most important tissues and organs at cost to the less important areas. It is essential to understand that this mechanism is a life-preserving one and makes sense within the concept of survival. We can afford to have our skin compromised up to a certain degree. The body will "use up its credit" in this area before a more important organ will be asked to give up some of its function. During healing, this means that vital organs such as the brain or the heart will clear of symptoms first,

---

30 Vithoulkas, G. The Science of Homeopathy, Grove Press: New York, 1980

before the less important organs such as the skin return to normal. In homeopathic and naturopathic thought, this phenomenon is referred to as the Hierarchy of Organs. It is my belief that this hierarchy goes hand in hand with the development of miasms. The first miasm shows only a relatively shallow depth of disease on this hierarchical scale, whereas the last miasm displays the deepest disease states and the most life-threatening afflictions. In between, we see a logical progression along the vital importance of the organs and tissues affected.

Keeping the idea of a hierarchy of disease progression in mind, we will now look at a naturopathic scenario of events describing the onset of chronic disease.

Digestion

In the first instance, early settler probably suffered from digestive disorders. A change to a diet with a completely different type of fibre (cereal husks instead of vegetable peels) would have had an irritating effect on the digestive mucosa. Lectins (see above) would have added to this process. The mucosa would have tried to protect itself by secreting extra mucus, which then had the effect of slowing down the absorption of nutrients. The irritation by foreign fibre can also cause diarrhoea whereas eating a diet with lower water content (cereals instead of vegetables/fruit) would have had a constipating effect. All these are common Psoric symptoms.

Being exposed to a critical mass of ingestible moulds, parasites and germs would in the first instance have also affected the gut and caused acute as well as chronic digestive problems. Once parasites have got a foothold they are difficult to get rid of if the environment is favourable. We know that a diet high in cereals predisposes us to developing unfavourable bowel flora. This in turn can invite parasites such as worms and Candida. The only way to get rid of these permanently is to include the removal of cereals from our diet into a therapeutic programme. Early man did not have this option and of course did not see the connection. Nowadays we are aware of the connection, but we chose not to take any notice, because our problems are not so obviously situated in the digestive system anymore. And so we fool ourselves that it would not make a difference.

Liver and Kidney

The next area affected by physical disease would have been the liver as all blood coming from the intestines in the first instance passes through the liver. If the intestinal mucosa became irritated and compromised, it would have let through a more than average amount of substances that were not designed to pass to the liver. This means that the liver would have had more work to do than before and in turn became compromised and sluggish. Portal stasis is the technical term for this state.

Lucky for the early settler, this was all at still a very mild level. And humans are very resilient. If they were not, how could we have survived millennia of abuse?

However, once the liver is compromised, the kidneys follow. A diet much lower in water content would have strained the kidneys in the long run. This is because metabolic poisons would have been passing through in higher concentrations increasing the risk of damage to kidney tissues. The diet also left higher acid levels in the body which need to be eliminated by the kidneys, again causing them to work harder and perhaps be damaged. As homeopaths we can begin to recognise certain Psoric remedies – first Calcarea and Sulphur, now Lycopodium.

Respiratory and Skin

Bowel, liver and kidneys are all important elimination organs. If all three major elimination organs are too busy, we build up a backlog of wastes. Our blood and lymph become slow and thick and we generally feel sluggish and tired. We begin eliminating extra waste (from endogenous waste and acid-forming foods) through our lungs and may therefore begin suffering from respiratory complaints. We also may begin trying to get rid of extra waste through our skin and may therefore begin suffering from skin rashes and lesions. Our skin ph would have changed by now to provide a beautiful breeding ground for mites.

Allergy

Alternative medicine has often claimed that food allergies are due to a "leaky gut".[31]

The idea is that the gut walls become irritated, inflamed and eventually more porous, letting through partially digested food items which the systemic immune system needed to mop up. Part of this systemic immune reaction was the release of either histamine or other inflammatory substances which then caused symptoms in any part of the body.

Luckily, we are in some way protected from serious harm due to this process. We possess an antibody located along our gut walls called IgA which attaches to the particles and marks them for phagocytosis, i.e. to be eaten up and dissembled. This is a normal, non-pathological body-process.

31 Krantz BA, Melnyk RA, Zhang S, et al. A phenylalanine clamp catalyzes protein translocation through the anthrax toxin pore. Science. 2005; 309 (5735):777-81

However, if too many undesirable food particles are detected (as dietary lectins and other pathogenic substances increase) the IgA mechanism becomes overworked and cannot keep up. In this case some particles will escape into lymph tissue or blood and stimulate other antibodies (IgG and IgE) into action.

In the Psoric individual, who at first did not necessarily have majorly irritated or inflamed gut walls, more and more lectins, gliadin and other large particles from food may have routinely escaped the IgA guard and subsequently activated IgG and/or IgE antibodies. The more grains were eaten, the more substances escaped, and the more likely it was that IgG/IgE became involved. The difference between IgA and IgG/IgE is that IgA acts locally in the gut and does not cause systemic histamine release nor systemic inflammation, but IgG/IgE do.[32] In essence, the more grains were eaten, the more inflammation and histamine release became a common feature, anywhere in the body.[33]

As it happens Psora is allergic, and many homeopaths consider Psora to be the base miasm for hay fever. In line with this idea, what is Psora allergic to? Hay! Grass! Could it be that eating cereals has caused a layer of allergy in all human beings, an allergy that is so subtle and nowadays so removed from the digestive system (through suppression over the course of 10 millenia) that we simply have not got a clue where it came from? Open your eyes and your mind to this possibility. Many nutritionists swear that eating wheat products may cause any symptom under the sun. Many homeopaths dismiss this as ridiculous and faddy. But

32 Liska D, Bland J. Digestion and Excretion. Functional Medicine, chapter 17: p 193-194

33 Hunter JO. Food allergy – or enterometabolic disorder? Lancet.1991; 338 (8765):495-96

we should know better. We are the ones who say that suppression moves symptoms deeper.

Nobody is suggesting that avoiding cereals will cure all disease, but for now please keep an open mind to the idea that cereals are a contributing factor to chronic disease. As we said before, chronic disease needs susceptibility as well as a disease stimulus. And the stimulus is multi-factorial. So cereals are only part of the story. But if you want to achieve a complete cure you must avoid cereals as they are part of the stimulus. Then you must identify the other stimuli and avoid these too. Eating cereals on a daily basis and in large amounts is a maintaining cause. Always and without exception. This is because homo sapiens is poorly adapted to their consumption.[34]

On the physical level, Psora is superficial in that no organ or system was pathologically damaged. All that happened at this stage was a general slowing down, digestive irritation and sluggish elimination. Is it possible to die from a purely Psoric complaint? Perhaps. For instance it may be possible that the thyroid gland becomes underactive to such a degree (without tissue damage) that life cannot be sustained. But in essence we are still dealing with a slowing down and not with a malignancy or a destructive process.

Psoric Disease Stimuli

In the case of Psora, we have identified cereals, alcohol, lack of aerobic exercise, exposure to a critical mass of parasites

34 In fact, we have a gene for gluten intolerance. Many of us have this gene switched on and eating even the smallest amount of gluten, as much as a pinhead, will set in motion an auto-immune cascade that lasts for months, possibly years. We can tolerate a small amount because we are very resilient and able to adapt to some degree, but we do not know how large or small this amount is for the individual. Nowadays, the threshold tolerance level depends of course on how otherwise weakened the individual's system is. More about this later.

and germs as stimuli. The Psoric susceptibility is anxiety. Anxiety about survival caused the behaviour (settling down and growing crops) which stimulated physical Psora into being. Depression and despair are a result of Psora and can be seen as mental/emotional symptoms of it, just as scabies is a physical symptom of Psora.

Intermittent anxiety alone does not make anyone ill if they eat a health maintaining diet, get enough exercise, do not abuse drugs or alcohol and do not expose themselves to a critical mass of pollution and germs. The problem is that anxiety will almost always cause compensatory health-eroding behaviours which then act as stimuli for physical chronic disease. But if it were possible to avoid the negative behaviour, perhaps physical disease would never happen.

Of course we must remember that nowadays, avoiding Psoric disease stimuli will not cure. This is because our bodies (not the structure of our DNA) have adapted and got stuck in a Psoric state so that we will express Psora even without stimuli, although in a much milder way. (Similarly, and complicating the issue, our bodies are also stuck in all other four miasmatic states, all with their own disease stimuli.) But this is where our nosodes and polycrests come in and can get us unstuck. Once all disease stimuli have been removed, anti-Psoric nosodes and polycrests may do the rest.

What we need to recognise is that continuing to indulge in Psoric stimuli will bring on Psora again and again in the way of a maintaining cause, even if we take homeopathic remedies to reduce the Psoric taint. Avoiding the stimuli as well as using homeopathy to get out of the Psoric state will facilitate a significant improvement in health.

If we believe that a good homeopathic prescription will take away the susceptibility to Psora and therefore the stimuli will not act as a trigger anymore, we are mistaken. If we look at this in detail we will see that the homeopathic remedy will take days if not weeks to take away the susceptibility, ie complete the healing. Meanwhile, if the exposure to triggers is on-going, the remedy will not yet have had time to complete the healing and Psora will be triggered all over.

So what about the instances of healing that do take place with homeopathy alone? I believe these are healings of states that are so relatively extreme, or indeed relatively contained, that all we see is return to the nowadays normal state of health for the person's age and circumstances. But this is not a cure of chronic disease. The person will sooner or later be affected by something else, because we have not removed the triggers. We have just reduced the tendency to be affected by the triggers in a certain way. For instance, if we cure somebody of a constant back-ground headache that had been present for 3 months, this is of course a wonderful relief for the patient. But it does not protect her from chronic disease for the rest of her life, even if the headache remedy was a deep-acting miasmatic remedy such as Natrum muriaticum for instance. What I suspect has taken place is an eradication of the emotional trigger and a reduction in her susceptibility to this emotional trigger. But she is not now protected from heart disease, or from chemical toxins affecting her. Whether and when she will fall ill from something else will all depend on her life-style and her hidden susceptibilities. If you do not agree with me at this point, please bear with me, I will come back to this issue at the end of the miasmatic road. Hopefully it will make sense to you then.

The Benefits of Psora

The agricultural revolution brought man a safer and more civilised life. The problems of food supply and shelter were solved, and this was a tremendous improvement for mankind. But the price was high. Man became subject to chronic disease. First signs were seen in the digestive system, on the skin, and in mild irritation and allergy of the respiratory system (of course not recognised as allergy). These problems never properly resolved, not because a scratch mite had infected man, but because man remained in a situation where his behaviour continuously stimulated Psoric complaints. Less exercise, less suitable nutrition, poor sanitation and chronic low-level anxiety maintained his behaviour over many generations and with this chronic disease. The scratch mite had a field day on such a terrain. Fortunately – with the help of salt, sulphur, and herbal lotions and potions – man found ways of suppressing scabies, and this enabled the story of social evolution to carry on. Without suppression of scabies, man and woman would have been most unattractive to look at and probably would have spent more time scratching than in pursuit of the opposite sex.

Even if man had had a true (educated) choice in the matter, he would have been happy to pay the price because he gained a safer, more peaceful life, with a potential. Because once his most basic needs were met he had spare time and energy to turn to higher goals such as mechanical inventions and academia. And this he certainly did.

Epigenetics

The science of epigenetics[35] is investigating the influence of environmental factors on our gene expression. Our genetic material has the ability to be switched on and off in sections. This causes a change in how our body functions, looks, responds etc. Certain environmental factors have been identified to change the expression of our DNA. In the individual this switch may remain permanent or may be reversed. Epigenetics have found some very tentative evidence of dietary changes having an epigenetic influence on not only the individual, but also the next generation and the following one too. Equally, epigenetics has identified the pathway by which cocaine changes our DNA expression to "addictive" type. This change remains long after exposure. If addiction could be transferred to the next generation in the same way as dietary influences might be, descendants would be in the "addictive" state even if they never indulged. This does sound remarkably like a miasm in action.

Could it be possible that a prolonged exposure to Psoric stimuli in early man caused a number of changes in our DNA expression which now permanently causes us to be ill in a Psoric way? And could it be that this change in our DNA expression could be reversed by giving anti-miasmatic treatment plus avoiding the maintaining Psoric disease stimuli?

Up and Beyond Psora

The story of social evolution carries on beyond Psora and the agricultural revolution. And with it the story of chronic disease unravels. As homeopaths, we recognise that chronic

35 http://epigenome.eu/ 13th Jan 2012

disease deepened, and we have blamed this on further invincible infections. This view does not serve us anymore. We realise now that infection is the result of a weakened state and not the cause of it.

As we discussed earlier, Psoric symptoms seemed to have developed in a certain order that is reminiscent of the homeopathic theory of the hierarchy of organs. This order and the reverse of it as stated in the Law of Cure implies that the body is intelligent in its survival mechanisms. Vital body parts are allowed to become affected by disease only after less vital parts have been compromised to saturation level. Further compromise would lead to death of the part and therefore death of the whole organism. So only when a less important organ has used up all its credit, another, slightly more important part will begin doing so. In effect this means that the less important organ saves the more important organs from damage. We could call it a sacrifice that must be made in order to spare the whole organism from damage or death. When our skin is affected by acne, this is far preferable than if our lungs were affected by similar bacterial infection and inflammation. The skin takes the pressure and the lungs are spared. We can live with inflammation on the skin (to some degree), but our lungs must be free to breathe easily without inflammation. Most homeopaths would be very familiar with this idea, but perhaps not with the parallel found in the evolution of miasms.

Just as with symptoms in the individual person, the miasmatic affliction of the human race happened along similar laws. The first miasm, Psora, gradually spreading amongst the earth's population and becoming stronger as generations passed, in effect made a sacrifice of the collective state of health of the human species in order for social progress to happen. But had this sacrifice not been made and had homo sapiens remained in his ecological niche as a hunter-gatherer, most of the human population may have become extinct (due to food shortage). Also, social evolution would not have taken place.

Psora saved humanity from remaining bound too closely to the natural food-chain. It enabled the human population to expand beyond what the original food-chain and eco-system could support. It allowed humanity to burst free from nature's chains and rise above the rest of all that moved and breathed.

We paid the price with a permanent deterioration in our state of health. But this was marginal at first and no-one took any notice.

The Story of Chronic Disease in a Nutshell

There was one flaw that kicked off the process of chronic disease. This flaw was simply being human as opposed to animal. After this our collective life-force tried to heal the consequences of being human by coming up with several options in succession. But unfortunately it never succeeded. All that happened was social progress of the species on the one hand and physical/mental/emotional decline of the individual on the other.

Parallel to Psora

Going back to hunter gatherer, we remember that the world had become a threatening place and that food was becoming scarce due to growing populations. Pre-Psoric man had chosen to solve this problem by growing his own food and settling down. He was driven by his anxiety.

But if we observe carefully we find that the problem of security of food and shelter can be solved by taking an alternative path.

The Life Of A Nomad

Much sooner than full blown Psora, but at the same time as Psoric susceptibility emerged in the millennia before the agricultural revolution, man left Africa. Or better – *some* left Africa. Little by little and generation by generation they covered the ground until even South America was populated. We do not know whether another hominid species lived in South America, but we do know that Europe and parts of Asia were already populated by other hominids such as Neanderthal.

This type of travelling person must necessarily have been less anxious and more daring.

Moving on to cover the rising demand in food supply is certainly an obvious solution. At first it may seem less innovative than settling down and growing crops, a totally unheard of activity. But at second glance, it shows an equally valid and definitely more courageous attitude.

Man on the move thought he had it all worked out. But wherever he turned, people were already there! And these people were better hunters. Neanderthal was an apex predator with a larger brain than homo sapiens. Ferocious and adapted to his surroundings, he had the advantage – at first. I imagine there were many clashes whilst homo sapiens was on the move to expand his territory. This daring and adventurous type therefore needed to work on his defensive and probably offensive skills. He had to become pronouncedly aggressive in order to stand a chance.

The second peril was winter. Homo sapiens had arrived in the temperate zone and even tried to move further north, way into the Arctic Circle. But now he was subject to the seasons. Poor hunting and gathering in the winter made life difficult, especially with Neanderthal living in the cave next door.

Even if this type of man wanted to settle down, the seasons and competition for hunting grounds prevented him from doing so. He remained nomadic moving from one place to another, but probably within a territory, however large it may have been.

How did nomad eventually solve his problem of securing a non-problematic food supply?

He noticed that some animals were rather docile and easier to catch than others. These could be kept and bred for food purposes. If you could not hunt all year round, why not catch/breed your own animal and keep it for the winter?

And so we witness the emergence of another miasm – Tuberculosis[36].

Animal Husbandry

Nomads were necessarily more daring. They encountered many difficult situations on the way. They had to hunt different types of prey, stand up to indigenous tribes and brave previously unknown weather conditions. A spirit of bravery and aggression had to be transmitted from generation to generation in order to make survival possible. These people were obviously quite different in their make-up to those who settled down to grow grains in hot climates.

Nomads had to move around in order to find greener pastures as the feeding of their herd animals was paramount to

---

36 In reality, animal husbandry was also practiced in the fertile crescent by early settlers and local nomads alike. There is therefore no true split into settler/Psora and nomad/Tuberculosis. But I believe that presenting these two miasms in this extreme and schema-like way will help us understand the evolution of miasms.

their survival. This made change and adventure a normal way of life. A degree of fearlessness and ignorance of danger had to be cultivated in order to not only survive but make the most of this kind of life. Desire for change, fearlessness, aggression, adventure. Which miasm does this remind us of?

There is more – a nomad's life was much less busy than a hunter-gatherer's. Hunting was almost unnecessary. This saved a lot of time. The animal herds were quickly checked, especially by the time nomad had also learnt to use horses and other animals to ride on. Newly trained wolf cubs[37] did the rounding up and kept watch all day and night. This brought considerable relief to survival anxiety as a good night's rest was finally possible. After all, a wolf's hearing and sense of smell is so much more acute than a human's.

The Male Nomad

The male nomad attended the animal herds.

For the rest of the day, the men folk were more or less idle, unless there was some slaughtering to do, or maybe mending tents and making tools which would not be taking place every day. Physical labour was therefore much reduced.

In the first instance this was a considerable advantage and allowed nomad to breathe easier. But similar to Psora, it brought with it some very negative physiological effects

---

37 Man's best friend: Wolves were the greatest threat to early nomad living in temperate zones. They were omnipresent, hunted in packs and dragged away children and herd animals. So what did early nomad do to solve his problem? The opposite of what you expect, of course, in true tubercular fashion! He managed to tame wolf cubs and make them his best friend. They protected him from wild beasts and helped him round up his precious herds. And so we witness tubercular reverse psychology in its first and original form.

on body statistics and endorphins. Man was lacking good-mood hormones.

Our male nomad suddenly had considerable stretches of time to do ... nothing. Life had become less threatening, but now a new sensation set in. Boredom.

Boredom and lack of endorphins are a bad combination. Both were only mild, but nevertheless were part of the problem that triggered a compensatory behaviour which turned out to be one of our disease stimuli for the Tubercular miasm.

How did nomad escape his boredom and bad mood? Instead of becoming depressed and slow like his Psoric cousin, he did more of what he had cultivated in the last millennia and what had helped him to establish his advantage – he became more adventurous, more daring, and more aggressive. Much testosterone and adrenalin based activity was now engaged in, all just to satisfy the need for entertainment and to keep boredom at bay. Welcome past-times were games on horseback as well as festivities. I imagine that bravery, competition and even cruelty were common traits amongst these people. One such activity where young men could prove themselves was perhaps attacking other tribes and raping and stealing their women-folk and bringing home on horseback anything that could be carried away: animals, animal skins, tools, weapons and household goods. It is my conviction that whereas Psora was mostly peaceful, Tuberculosis set the scene for cruelty as a way of stimulation.

In the nomad male then, periods of quiet and boredom brought on restlessness and frustration which drove him on to invent and engage in games and entertainments. And occasionally he would find an outlet in aggressive behaviour towards other tribes and even settlers.

I believe that this pattern of seesawing between boredom and adrenaline-based activities strained the male's system by a minor but nevertheless considerable degree. In particular, the adrenal glands would have suffered[38] as they are majorly involved in mediating the stress response. By being asked to produce much adrenalin and cortisol repeatedly at stressful but exciting times, they became fatigued and strained, because in spite of long stretches of boredom, nomad's adrenal energy resources and cell components never got the chance to recover completely due to other factors (discussed below) that were a feature of his new lifestyle. Eventually, the scales were tipped towards chronic disease.

The Female Nomad

The story for nomad women was slightly different. Labour division was firmly established but this was something relatively new. Early hunter-gatherers before Psora did not have labour division. But now, after the social evolution to animal husbandry, long hunts were off and women got far less exercise than ever before. They still walked during gathering of fruit and vegetables, and looking after the children kept them on their feet, but long hunts at jogging speed were not necessary.

Their daily duties revolved around gathering, preparing food, general household (tent) duties and caring for the children. Milking, making cheese and yoghurt as well as preparing meals was a simple but time-consuming matter.

---

38 Wilson, JL. Adrenal fatigue, the 21st century stress syndrome. Petaluma: Smart Publications; 2001

Keeping the tents in order and in good repair as well as making clothes and tools was also on the agenda. I believe that nomad woman had a busier life than her male counterpart. This helped her to feel less bored, although to some degree she would also have suffered from bad moods. This is because she got less exercise than her hunter ancestor and so had lower levels of endorphins to keep her happy. Perhaps there was also a feeling of frustration because she was not allowed to join in the general merry-making on horseback. And was there even some resentment and feeling of being restrained and prevented from running free as her male companions were able to do all day long?

Nomad woman became bad tempered and only truly happy when feast days allowed her to dance and temporarily forget her heavy chains and chores. I also believe that she compensated for her frustration by engaging in pretty much the only outlets she had that were socially acceptable – eating, gossiping and arguing.

Thus the daily life of nomad woman was busy but burdensome for her. She felt bogged down and only physical exertion made her feel better. She did not engage in the same seesaw pattern as the male, but was still affected by her negative state of mind, over-eating and the other factors that came along with the change to animal husbandry. These factors were powerful enough to bring on chronic disease, as we will see.

Tubercular Attitude

Early nomad depended on his tribe to provide shelter, security and nourishment. This is why we see in the tubercular personality a strong need to be in company. In addition, social evolution had bestowed him and her with a high-spirited nature and an adventurous and daring temperament. Both sexes were in essence gregarious and fun-loving, always up for a game and a show. Unfortunately, as we will see below, the rest of their life-style did not allow the male to sustain the kind of adrenalin-depleting pattern we described above. What ensued was a cycle of addiction swinging from periods of high activity to near burn out. Much the same as seen in Phosphorus, a key Tubercular remedy.

The female nomad, in contrast, was not allowed to express her high-spirited nature. She became bogged down, frustrated and bad tempered, finding outlet only on feast days and by overeating. Mrs Sepia was born.

These attitudes and behaviour alone would have depleted both sexes mildly but not enough to bring on chronic disease in a miasmatic way. If both male and female would have been able to rest, exercise properly and replenish their resources on all levels, they would have remained healthy and strong. After all homo sapiens was designed to withstand a long life of hunting and gathering, defending against the elements and wild beasts. As long as he remained true to his design. But as we know, intermittent survival anxiety had driven him on to find solutions and liberate him from his struggle against the elements. Whilst animal husbandry provided such a solution for the human species, it opened the door to chronic disease coupled with a new set of mental/emotional problems – boredom, frustration and aggression.

Let us now look at the more physical factors that brought on Tuberculosis, the miasm.

Tuberculosis, the disease

Tuberculosis is transmitted to humans through infected milk and meat, and between humans by droplet transmission (sneezing, coughing etc), i.e. close and repeated body contact. Crowded and unsanitary living conditions would favour the spread of this disease, just as that of any. Until the advent of modern pharmaceuticals, tuberculosis was kept under control by exposure to sunlight and fresh air.

A wild herd-animal infected with tuberculosis would have recovered or died, infecting several others of its herd, depending on factors such as proximity, frequency of contact and inherent weakness. The likelihood of a human hunter eating the meat of such an animal was low. If it happened, the hunter's immune system would have had to be susceptible in order to fall prey to such a deadly illness. In many of those rare cases of infection, probably in up to 80% or so, the disease did not fall on favourable soil (I am speculating of course). In the rest of cases it did. To become latent and miasmatic, however, the disease energy must have been (as we saw in the case of Psora/scabies) a match for early humans' susceptibility; and not just for the individual but for the human species as such.[39]

So how did the human species acquire the Tubercular miasm?

Let us remember that a miasm comes into being just as any disease, but on a collective scale and over a long period of time. We need to see a marriage of susceptibility with stimulus. The Tubercular susceptibility was a collective attitude which must have been seen as advantageous by

---

39 To remind yourself of my reasoning, see "Susceptibility and Disease Stimulus" on page 13 and "Attitude, Behaviour and Chronic Disease" on page 18

a critical mass of individuals. This attitude must also have been present for many generations in order to bring about a matching behaviour that could have functioned as a trigger/disease stimulus. The behaviour must also have been maintained over many generations in order to provide sufficient cover and in order for the disease picture to become firmly and collectively established. A single incident of acute disease does not trigger a miasmatic layer of disease in all of mankind; it takes much more than that. It must have been a true energetic marriage (simillimum) of attitude with behaviour, maintained over many generations and prevalent in a critical mass of people.

We have established that acute infection with tuberculosis was not this disease stimulus that we are looking for. Tuberculosis is an infection which in about 22% of cases leads to death. The symptoms are severe, drawn out and cause much suffering to the victim. This suffering is and was no match with the intermittent anxiety as susceptibility of early man as described above. Intermittent anxiety as an attitude is not strong enough to marry with a deadly disease. It would be like killing house spiders with nuclear bombs.

It follows that widespread trans-generational (miasmatic) tubercular infection in humans did not take place while humans were hunter gatherers and susceptible to acute disease only. There must have been something else that changed before a terrible disease such as tuberculosis could take hold on a collective and chronic scale.

Cross-Infection

A herd animal kept by nomads would have been considerably restricted in its movements for some of its daily life so that proximity and frequency of contact with other animals was increased. This way, disease incidence would have also increased. I suppose that at that time tuberculosis in wild herd animals was probably as common as any acute disease in humans. It did not become chronic in the sense of a miasm until herd animals were domesticated and subject to similar restrictions, anxieties and changes that man was experiencing.

As humans were now living off the meat and milk of such animals, not being aware of the infection until the animal was near its end, tuberculosis would have spread more readily to them than to hunter-gatherers. Whether they fell victim or not depended, as we know, on their susceptibility and on a critical mass of germs attacking. This naturally reduced the incidence of acute infection.

Also, humans could not become infected from latent tuberculosis in animals (or other humans). Infection took place only whilst the disease was in its acute state, again reducing its incidence in humans. This is another reason why other factors besides infection must have been present to bring about a miasmatic layer of disease.

What are these other factors?

Dairy

Apart from the change in attitude described above and the ensuing seesawing from high activity to burn out, there was a considerable change in diet. Dairy products were added and became a mainstay of the daily diet, especially in the winter. Gathering still took place, subject to seasons, and probably also some hunting, but much reduced.

Dairy products such as yoghurt and cheese could be produced all year round and therefore provided early nomad with a practical solution to his survival issues in temperate climates. Whilst protein, fat and calcium needs were covered by these innovative food items they nevertheless had and still have several downsides.

Dairy Intolerance

Before we go into detail, let us discuss a common misconception about the ability to digest dairy.

After the age of four, humans are genetically programmed to lose the ability to digest milk sugar (lactose). The gene that is responsible for the production of the enzyme that breaks down milk sugar turns itself "off".[40] It has now been established that early Europeans as far back as 5000 BC did not have the ability to digest milk sugar.[41] The original setting was the "off" setting, i.e. no milk please.[42]

Regardless of present day settings of this gene, early nomad living well before 5000 BC had this gene turned off, making him intolerant to dairy – at least in his digestive system. Common symptoms would have been irritated mucous membranes of the digestive tract, mucus in stool,

40 Beja-Pereira, et al. Gene-culture coevolution between cattle milk protein genes and human lactase genes. Nature Genetics, 2003; 35(4), 311-313.

Enattah, N.S. et al. Identification of a variant associated with adult-type hypolactasia. Nature Genetics, 2002; 30(2), 233-237.

Lomer, M.C.E.,et al. Review article: lactose intolerance in clinical practice – myths and realities. Alimentary Pharmacology & Therapeutics, 2008; 27 (2),

41 Bersaglieri, T.,et al. Genetic signatures of strong recent positive selection at the lactase gene. American Journal of Human Genetics, 2004; 74(6), 1111-1120.

Jobling, M.A., et al. Human Evolutionary Genetics: origins, peoples and disease. London/New York, 2004.

42 The question is whether this gene can be and is/was turned on at some point to make dairy digestion possible without collateral damage. Some researchers claim that presently only 5% of adults have the gene turned off, making them intolerant of dairy. Others claim that all adults have this gene turned off, making everyone intolerant of dairy foods. The truth is probably somewhere in between.

gas, bloating, cramps and diarrhoea. Incidentally all common Phosphorus symptoms.

Before early nomad managed to turn his dairy digestion gene to the "on" setting on a collective scale (if he ever did), several hundred or perhaps a thousands of years passed. His constitution weakened by the constant irritation in his guts, other factors such as infection and mental/emotional anxieties were more likely to make a critical difference. As we will see, much happened to early nomad's constitution during those millennia of gas and spluttering.

So let us discuss the problems with dairy foods in more detail.

Acidity

Just as with cereals, some dairy products leave an acidic ash in our bodies. (For reasons why this is disadvantageous, see above). If balanced by alkaline-providing foods this is not a problem. But for early nomad, alkaline foods were scarce for at least 3-5 months of the year, i.e. during the colder seasons. During these colder months dairy and meat were probably making up 75% or more of the daily diet. Even with milk and yoghurt as neutral foods, i.e. leaving neither alkaline nor acidic ash, probably something like 50% of the daily diet was acid-producing, 25% neutral and 25% alkaline. Sustained over months this can easily lead to acid-elimination symptoms such as catarrh and phlegm production in respiratory and digestive systems. Yes – the common cold.

Mineral Imbalances

Over-consumption of dairy as practised by early nomad produced an imbalance of minerals in several ways.

First, in most if not all individuals dairy produce caused a slight irritation of the mucus membranes in the digestive system due to the lectins contained in dairy foods.[43] This was confounded by the acid/alkaline imbalance described above. Once the digestive membranes were irritated, the process of nutrient absorption became impaired. In early nomad this effect would have been only mild, but nevertheless present.

Second, the dietary balance of calcium to magnesium required for humans is 2:1 (Ca:Mg). But cow's milk has a Ca:Mg ratio of 10:1, and cow's cheese about 28:1. Even if early nomad did not live on milk from cattle but from goats and sheep, the ratio would have still been too high in favour of calcium. Eating a lot of dairy would therefore not have provided man with enough magnesium compared to calcium. Other minerals such as zinc, chromium and manganese are also in poor supply compared to vegetables that hunter-gatherer had as a staple food.

Third, the absorption of calcium across the digestive membrane is conducted by the same pumps as that of some of the other minerals. And the body is programmed to favour calcium over the other minerals, i.e. it always takes calcium first before it considers the others. If you eat a diet too high in calcium you will therefore absorb plenty of it, but not much of the other minerals. By the time the pumps are disengaged to turn their attention to magnesium, zinc, etc., much of the food/nutrients will have travelled too far down the alimentary canal and be lost in stool.

---

43 These lectins cause similar problems to the lectins contained in pulses and grains, see "Lectins" on page 30, within Psora.

If dairy is eaten only occasionally, these effects will be diluted beyond relevance. But for early nomad dairy was a staple food that dominated every meal.

In this way, early nomad – certainly for 3-5 months of the year – built up a deficiency in minerals. I doubt whether he was able to make good this deficiency in the warmer months. My suspicion is that once he got used to eating a lot of dairy, he continued even in the warmer months. This is because dairy has a certain addictive quality due to opiate compounds contained in it.[44] Once you are used to eating cheese and yoghurt, you will continue.

Phosphorus and Vitamin D

Cheese contains a lot of phosphorus. Early nomad would have been supplied with a disproportionate amount of it, much more than a hunter-gatherer would have eaten. As it happens, Phosphorus is a key Tubercular polycrest.

High phosphorus levels impair the conversion of vitamin D into its active form.[45] Vitamin D is important for immune function and it is initially produced by exposure of skin to natural daylight (before it is activated in the liver and kidneys).

Early nomad was subject to three factors which reduced his vitamin D levels and therefore impaired his immunity – compared to hunter-gatherer he ate a diet much higher in phosphorus; he spent six months of the year in less daylight; he had to wear more clothing to keep warm for a

---

44 Kitts DD, Weiler K. Bioactive proteins and peptides from food sources. Applications of bioprocesses used in isolation and recovery. Curr Pharm Des. 2003; 9(16):1309-23

   Teschemacher H. Opioid receptor ligands derived from food proteins. Curr Pharm Des. 2003; 9(16):1331-44

45 http://lpi.oregonstate.edu/infocenter/minerals/phosphorus/14th Jan 2012

substantial amount of months thereby reducing his surface exposure to sunlight dramatically.

Tuberculosis and other infections of the respiratory system are most common during the colder months. And a relative deficiency of Vitamin D is probably one of the contributing factors.

Inflammation and Arachidonic Acid

Another disadvantage of a diet too high in dairy foods (without the balancing presence of enough vegetables and fruit) is its ability to promote inflammation in general. Inflammation is an important immune process promoted by prostaglandins made from arachidonic acid (AA – an omega 6 fatty acid). Problems start when there is either too much AA, or if it is not balanced by omega 3 fatty acids. Unfortunately dairy is low in omega 3 and high in omega 6, especially AA. It follows that a diet that relies heavily on dairy foods promotes inflammation.[46]

Early nomad would therefore have been prone to inflammation which was mostly expressed on his gut membranes, but also on his upper and lower respiratory membranes (see below "allergy") and his skin.

As homeopaths we recognise inflammation of the superficial membranes of our body as the hallmark of the Tubercular miasm. The outer skin as well as all the respiratory and digestive membranes are affected in this manner producing eczema, asthma, chest infections and digestive complaints (diarrhoea).

---

46 Seaman DR. The diet-induced proinflammatory state: a cause of chronic pain and other degenerative diseases? J Manipulative Physiol Therapy. 2002; 25:168-79.

Vasquez A. Reducing pain and Inflammation naturally. Part 2: New insights into fatty acid supplementation and its effect on eicosanoid production and genetic expression. Nutritional Perspectives. 2005; January:5-16

AA is also present in meat, and nowadays meat, dairy and plant seed oils are major sources of this inflammation promoting substance. Hunter-gatherer, who ate a lot of meat was also taking in a lot AA. But in those days the composition of animal fat was different. It was very much higher in omega 3 and much lower in saturated and omega 6 than it is now.[47] Any AA hunter-gatherer ate was therefore balanced regularly and sufficiently by omega 3. But the meat of a domesticated animal, even that of a semi-wild herd animal, is low in omega 3.

In addition to AA causing problems with inflammation, the slightly impaired state of nomad's adrenal glands caused imbalances in cortisol secretion. This confounds our problem further, as one of cortisol's roles is to keep inflammation in check.[48] Low cortisol equals high inflammation. Poor nomad was struck from both sides.

Allergy

The problem of the untoward inflammatory process is enormous. From the onset of the Tubercular miasm it has plagued man, producing ever more debilitating illnesses through the ages. Most medically named diseases are now recognised as having "inflammation" as a confounding

---

47 Cordain,L. et al. Fatty acid analysis of wild ruminant tissues: Evolutionary implications for reducing diet-related chronic disease. European Journal of Clinical Nutrition. 2002; 65:181-91

Crawford M.A. et al. Comparative studies on fatty acid composition of wild and domestic meat. Int J Biochem. 1970; 1:295-305

48 The adrenal glands are intimately involved in keeping inflammation to an appropriate level. Cortisol, a major stress hormone released by the adrenal glands, reduces inflammation and reduces histamine levels. This is a very important function, as without sufficient cortisol we produce inflammation and allergic symptoms. The effects can range from mildly bothersome as in mild hay fever to majorly limiting as in severe asthma. Adrenal fatigue can therefore have severe systemic consequences.

if not causative factor. These range from eczema, asthma, arthritis, infertility, ME to heart disease and cancer.

It is my belief that the process was put in motion in early nomad's time by the original imbalance of AA to omega 3, caused by a diet too high in dairy foods, as well as the over-taxing of the adrenals – causing disrupted cortisol secretion which hindered inflammation check.[49] Once early nomad's system had acquired this tendency to inflammation and continuously stimulated it by way of eating dairy as a maintaining cause, his system needed to react by eliminating on superficial levels such as through the airways, skin and digestive tract. I imagine he was displaying a more or less continuous mild "cold". Nowadays we would think of someone with a continuous cold as "allergic" to something. Hence the term allergic rhinitis. But in the case of early nomad there probably was no true allergy involving IgE antibodies, but just a never-ending inflammatory process affording continuous elimination.

Another intriguing detail is our Tubercular "allergy" to animal dander[50]. If we go back in time and imagine a nomad's tent we will see that during winter, man and animal lived in closer proximity than ever before in the history of mankind. Whereas dairy herd animals were kept outdoors, man's best friends – dog and horse – most probably were allowed to share shelter. Now imagine nomad's immune system switched into inflammatory mode as described above. Is it not plausible that it would also begin reacting to animal dander, especially of dog and horse? This

---

49 Munck A, Guyre PM, Holbrook NJ. Physiologic function of glucocorticoidsin stress and their relation to pharmacologic actions. Endocr rev. 1984; 5;2 5-44 Reichlin S. Neuroendocrine-immune interactions. N Engl J Med. 1993; 329(17): 146-53

50 Dander: skin flakes in an animal's fur or hair (cf dandruff)

would especially take place when his cortisol levels were intermittently too low to counteract histamine, the promoter of allergy. Histamine and cortisol balance each other in a way that cortisol blocks histamine. Impaired adrenal function as seen in early nomad would therefore promote allergy by this pathway too.

Early Nomad's Disease Process

The social evolution from hunter gatherer to nomad brought with it enormous advantages. Hunting became unnecessary and accidents and insecurities related to this activity ceased almost completely. Food was always available as long as the animals had enough to eat and survived the climate. Attacks from wild animals were much reduced due to domestication of wolves.

But just as early settler paid a price for solving his survival problems, early nomad did too. On the one hand he had a much higher exposure to infected animals and infected animal meat and milk. On the other hand his immune system was compromised by poorer nutritional content, physical crowding and poor hygiene (in tents) and lower exposure to sunlight. The diet induced a continuous low-level inflammatory state which became the hall-mark of the shift from acute to chronic disease.

A third factor affecting his health on a collective scale was the seesawing between high activity and burn out described above and for the females a continuous feeling of frustration, compensated for by overeating.

Of course, reproduction did its part to distribute any slight organ impairment evenly amongst the sexes of the progeny.

Addiction and the Adrenal Glands

What happened to the body of a nomad who spent long hours being bored, and relieving this with adrenalin and testosterone – based activities? I believe he entered a cycle of addiction. The quiet periods were unbearable to him. He got some relief from social entertainment, but also used sex, aggression and cruelty to stimulate himself into feeling "OK". Unfortunately his lifestyle did not allow for his system to truly replenish the nutritional and biochemical resources he used up during his extreme activity states. His adrenal glands would have been stimulated beyond their design and when he rested he became aware of a state of slight exhaustion beyond a normal tiredness. His reaction to this was to restart the cycle in order to feel "OK" again. In effect, nomad became addicted to adrenal stress. And his adrenal glands became more stressed as the years passed.

I believe that nowadays the Tubercular miasm is the base miasm for drug abuse for exactly the same reason, i.e. to relieve boredom out of a spirit for adventure and curiosity. The drugs used would be "uppers" such as cocaine. In contrast, the Psoric miasm is the base miasm for alcoholism to relieve depression.

A Curious Fact

Adrenal stress predisposes especially to one particular issue – chest weakness. Recurring chest infections, pneumonia and asthma are all commonly seen and linked to adrenal insufficiency, i.e. problems with cortisol output.[51] In other words, a person with adrenal insufficiency is more likely to suffer from chest and lung problems than someone whose adrenal glands are working well. The same is true

51 Wilson, JL. Adrenal Fatigue – the 21st century stress syndrome, Petaluma Smart Publications; 2001.

for eczema. Mothers who suffer from adrenal insufficiency have a higher risk of having offspring developing eczema soon after birth. The link is poor cortisol output causing unchecked inflammation.

Physical Tuberculosis

The physiological cycle of addiction to adrenal stress was not extreme from a collective point of view, although for the individual who overdid things it may have ended in poor immunity, burn out and death from respiratory disease. In this way tuberculosis was only one possible outcome for anyone living the Tubercular lifestyle and engaging in Tubercular behaviour (the disease stimulus).

But from a miasmatic angle the Tubercular miasm caused mostly superficial afflictions in the hierarchy or organs, in a way that many body parts became inflamed, but not damaged as in subsequent miasms.

Let us look at this more closely.

The digestive system would have suffered from chronic diarrhoea due to irritation of the mucosa by dairy. Continuous adrenal stimulation may have also added to increased gut activity almost in an IBS fashion.

The next organ affected would have been the liver, as we see in the Tubercular remedy Phosphorus, resulting in inflammation caused by too much saturated fat. The kidneys are next in line with additional salt (from cheese) having to be eliminated, leading to frequent urination, incontinence and enuresis, again very Tubercular symptoms.

Inflammation generally took hold of the membranes of the body (gut, respiratory, epidermis and synovial), causing diarrhoea, respiratory allergy, lung disease, eczema and arthritis.

Summary of Tuberculosis

The life of a nomad was considerably different from that of a hunter-gatherer. His daily activity levels were reduced leaving him idle and bored for long stretches of time. To compensate he began engaging in high adrenalin based activities which overtaxed his system and left him depleted. Dietary deficiencies and inflammation took toll, and exposure to a critical mass of germs and animal dander as well as poor supply of daylight and fresh air during the winter months.

His system became weakened and opened itself to chronic disease in Tubercular fashion. In spite of all this, early nomad was still quite healthy. He lived an outdoor life, with far more activity and exercise than most of us get now. His food was unadulterated and free of chemicals. Pure Tubercular miasm was therefore not such a bad state to be in – compared to what followed...

The Benefits of Tuberculosis, the Miasm

Animal husbandry solved the problem of food supply and gave protection from wild beasts in a most ingenious way. Humans benefitted tremendously and could breathe easier. Whereas Psora converted its spare energy into extending feelers into academic realms, Tuberculosis used a similar surplus for expanding its sheer enjoyment of life in more physical ways. The Tubercular miasm has enriched the human experience by encouraging us to be more daring, more adventurous, more fun-loving and gregarious. In essence it allows us to celebrate being alive. The fearless side of the miasm has enabled us to explore the world and break boundaries in physical ways. Thus the Tubercular miasm has been the driving force behind many marvellous accomplishments of the human species. And since only those who dare will succeed, the Tubercular miasm has its benefits still today.

The advantages of the Tubercular life-style were so tremendous that there was no way back. The susceptibility to Tuberculosis (intermittent survival anxiety) had been satisfied by adapting the animal husbandry life-style. The disease stimulus was the totality of factors (discussed above) associated with this. Tuberculosis – the disease – was not the cause of the Tubercular miasm, but the result of it. Tubercular problems were never resolved, not because our immune system was weakened by an invincible infection, but because man engaged in health eroding practices on a collective scale and over many generations. The behaviours became ingrained and could not be reversed as they were seen as advantageous. Not adapting those behaviours would have been a worse alternative.

On a collective scale, the Tubercular miasm saved the human species from extinction by solving the problem of food supply. By doing so, Tuberculosis moved man up the ladder of social evolution. Unfortunately, homo sapiens had to pay a price by descending into the realm of chronic disease.

Beyond Tuberculosis

Nomads have roamed the planet for millennia. But even in biblical times, i.e. 3,000 years BC they had begun mixing with settlers. Both groups adapted parts of their diet by exchanging goods for grains and pulses, and they stole or traded in women. For this reason, the distinction between Psora and Tuberculosis became blurred through the ages. Nowadays, the members of either group may express either miasm.

Whilst present-day 3rd world nomads and present-day 3rd world agricultural settlers will still be much healthier than the average westerner due to active outdoor lifestyles, limited suppression and relatively unadulterated nutrition, we nevertheless will see chronic conditions of Psoric and/or Tubercular nature. There may even be Sycotic or Syphilitic complaints depending on how much contact there is with urban settlers and on how far their mind and attitude has moved on from earlier miasms.

Psora and Tuberculosis both secured the food supply and freed up energy for higher purposes. In this way they fuelled social evolution.

But both miasms left the human species with new dilemmas.

The Psoric individual now found himself chronically anxious and depressed as well as sluggish and itchy on a physical level. The Tubercular person found himself swinging from exhaustion, boredom and frustration to excitement and aggression, with respiratory complaints and general inflammation becoming a common feature.

Both groups still had to spend hours performing physical labour. In addition, although the immediate need for food and shelter had been satisfied, they nevertheless were still subject to seasons, weather and other natural influences and factors they had absolutely no power or control over.

In this way, the intermittent anxiety had been exchanged for a less urgent, but omnipresent concern. This was still better than going back, but after a while man had enough. There had to be a way out of this eternal struggle and physical hardship.

What would man give to be free all day! Then he could finally enjoy himself and do exactly what he wanted....

Eventually we came up with a solution which would move us one step further away from nature and make us even less dependent on mother earth (we thought).

Urbanisation

6,000 years ago first cities had been established in the Middle East. These were large settlements built from stone buildings surrounded by strong walls to protect from attacks by nomadic tribes or other urban societies. The Old Testament is full of stories involving various urban settlements and our museums are well equipped with numerous artefacts and even parts of buildings bearing witness to early urban societies. Why these urban societies evolved exactly where they did has remained subject of much speculation.

What seems to have been accepted is that to support the population of such a city, a certain density of population in the surrounding countryside was required, as otherwise transport of daily provisions would have taken too long. After all, it was the local countryside population who was producing food for city dwellers.

By the same logic it is almost certain that large-scale hunter-gathering would have been out of fashion for many millennia and that agriculture and animal husbandry had been the norm for a long time. Obviously, hunting would not have produced enough provisions for a concentrated settlement of tens of thousands of people on a daily basis.

In our story of chronic disease and social evolution, urbanisation was the next step forward for society, but brought with it a further blow to our health. This is because it automatically divided the human species into those "providing" and those "provided for". Why would this matter?

To Have or To Have Not

For first city dwellers the question was not one of survival, but one of establishing themselves amongst the lucky few who could subsist on activities as far removed from physical labour as possible. This was the next step forward on the ladder of social evolution and brought about a class system or division between poor and rich. Obviously there had been poorer and richer and more junior and more senior nomads and settlers within each community, but urbanisation produced socially and miasmatically significant extremes way beyond what had existed before.

How did all this come about?

Cities probably arose out of the phenomena of trade and commerce. Nomads had been trading in food and goods for some time and trading routes were well established. Settlers welcomed friendly nomads, and mutually beneficial relationships were formed. Those settlements on well-trodden trade routes, near inexhaustible water sources and with better soil quality in the immediate environment did better than others. They soon expanded as nomads needed space to stay over night and had to make payments for this. Thus some settlers - and in turn nomads - were able to amass possessions beyond immediate need.

Over the centuries, man began exchanging goods and foods not just for immediate consumption, nor just to secure bare survival in the near future, but simply because he could. Underneath he still did it to satisfy his chronic survival anxiety that remained with him to this day, but on the surface he acquired far more than was useful or than he would ever need.

In addition, exchange of labour against goods was introduced and at some point money was invented. This was most significant in the evolution of society and miasms. It was now possible to divide labour beyond the division between husband and wife. Some people could cease growing crops or keeping animals and could do something they were perhaps more suited to or that they thought would bring them an easier life.

Class Society

The more Psoric individual had already begun shifting some of his energy into the realms of the mind. But now he could stop physical labour altogether and use his mental capacity to earn his living. This was timely as these newly emerging large settlements of very permanent nature needed to achieve some degree of organisation beyond a circle of elders sitting around a fire in the evenings. New professions such as teachers, scribes, lawyers, secretaries, town officials, and doctors emerged providing urban society with a rich variety of occupations and ways to gain respect.

Other individuals, of Psoric or Tubercular nature, adapted to urban life by establishing themselves in crafts such as carpentry, pottery and tailoring. They began exchanging food for their goods or later asked for money. In this way they supported the needs of the other urban dwellers whilst securing their own income.

A third group, probably the more Tubercular type, perhaps through sheer luck or by being quicker in recognising opportunities in these early days, began engaging in trade on a big scale. Strategic marriages and hierarchical command structures amongst and within trading clans/families slowly but surely increased their wealth and kept it securely within their hands.

A fourth group established itself as truly superior as its power was based on financial advantage backed up by land ownership and tradition/heritage. These were the descendants of Psoric settlers or Tubercular nomads of rank, i.e. the descendants of clan elders and chiefs. As their clans had been habitual occupants of stretches of land, in time they became landowners. Whether they lived in the cities or in the countryside, they turned all-powerful as the whole structure of society depended on the food the land could provide. I believe that land-ownership was seen as the most prestigious of these four new sections of society, and this is the section that transformed into what we now recognise as aristocracy. This group simply hung onto its legislative rights, probably because of traditional values as well as power and riches bestowed through ownership of land.

A fifth group remained behind and worked the fields and engaged in animal husbandry. As the other sections rose up, they lost personal power as they did not own the land they worked on and had nothing other to bargain with than their labour. But because of the sheer number of people in this position labour was worth very little, and eventually this group descended into the misery of serfdom. They never lived in the cities and so at first did not become "infected" by the newer miasms in a major way. This was advantageous from a health point of view, but otherwise very unfortunate.

Urban Life

Early urban life had one decisive measure of success – money. If you had enough, life was comfortable. You lived in some kind of permanent stone building, relatively secure against the elements and completely safe from wild animals. The male was the breadwinner and, depending on his class or the sector of society he belonged to, there was enough food, enough clothing and perhaps even some spare for newly emerging luxury articles. On top of this, again depending on your standing within society, you now had gained a measure of respect, at least over agricultural workers outside the city, but also over have-nots within. This was important to people now, as physical ways of maintaining hierarchy were lost.

But hierarchy maintains order and therefore it is intrinsically essential in any society. In hunter-gatherers times, and in our semi-human past, order was maintained through contests of physical strength. Whoever could wrestle down competition became alpha male, could chose females and rule the roost.

Urban society had left behind this kind of behaviour. Achieving status through belongings and wealth was now the order of the day. Physical strength was irrelevant although physical beauty was still relatively important in females. But even females were increasingly chosen for their connectedness and wealth and less for their childbearing ability and physical health.

Thus urban life was accompanied by completely altered values and priorities.

Have-nots were a sorry lot. Urban life produced many of this kind, living in squalor and misery, worse than any agricultural or nomadic society ever saw. Either having lost their ability to earn a living or having lost status, these individuals became the bottom of the heap. Criminal activity or begging was their only way of maintaining life as moving out to the countryside and beginning a life as a freeman or serf was impossible. There was simply no legal, or other, pathway for this.

In addition, attracted by the possibility of becoming "haves", some agricultural people relocated to cities and often just became lost in the anonymous urban underworld.

For the first time in the evolution of human societies, crime became one way to earn a living. Although nomads had engaged in robbery and rape, they did not do this exclusively, and not to survive. Most of the time they maintained their lives by peaceful animal husbandry. But in early urban societies (and in modern ones too) crime and begging became occupations just as any other.

Urban society therefore gave rise to many new opportunities and liberated much mental and creative energy to be diverted into progress. But it also brought about a new, distinct duality and interplay between poor and rich as well as good and evil.

The Physical Disadvantages of Urban Life

Man entered his urban phase of social evolution slightly weakened by Psora and Tuberculosis. In other words, there was a general sluggishness, a tendency to inflammation, nutrient deficiencies, as well as emotional taints beyond a general background anxiety such as mild depression, an inclination to alleviate frustration by engaging in cruelty or destruction, and a tendency to physiological and emotional addiction.

Whilst urbanisation gave man the option to reduce physical labour and free up energy to feed his desire for progress, it did nothing to cure his physical problems; quite the opposite. The gap between progress for society as a whole on the one side and physical health on the other became even wider.

Lack of Exercise

As physical strength became irrelevant for so many members of the more advantaged groups described above, physical exercise went out of fashion and was even frowned upon as it became associated with poorer groups who had to perform manual labour.

On a more immediate level, all living organisms are designed to reduce their energy expenditure to the bare minimum necessary for survival. And so we can hardly blame any early urban settlers for not going for their routine morning jog around the filthy urban streets.

The lower classes still got at least some exercise through their work, whether in their workshops or around the house. So it was mostly in the middle and upper classes that moving limbs beyond what was necessary for lifting drinks utensils or putting food into your own mouth became a rarity. Short walks or going up and down stairs was the maximum, but some noblemen engaged in popular games and hunts, giving them small opportunities for causing the heart to pump faster.

Rich women were the hardest hit as they literally had nothing to do. A complete lack of exercise led to a slowing down of metabolism, a negative change of blood and liver composition, sluggish lymph circulation and with it a back-log of endogenous waste elimination and wastes aggregating in tissues, weight gain and poor emotional balance. Rich men also experienced this, although probably to a lesser degree as they still had the benefits of hunting and games, or mild physical activity enforced by their business duties.

This very negative effect on body statistics was confounded by the deterioration of the diet in several significant ways.

Yeast and Mould

Whereas early settlers at first used mainly coarsely milled grains and water to prepare bread, soon man began leaving the dough out in the sun to ferment. This produced a softer texture and therefore a more desirable loaf. By Babylonian times and when urbanisation began, bread was leavened with sweet wine.

Whilst fermentation has some advantages such as enhancing of flavour, preservation and pre-digestion of foods, it also has a most significant disadvantage – its driving force is yeast. Yeast foods are generally rich in vitamin B, but this positive aspect is cancelled out by its many negative effects on human health.

Beyond yeast, early bakers did not realise that another relative of yeast was taking advantage of their lovely fare – mould! Modern bread making includes additives that prevent mould formation in bread, but in early urban days no such thing was available. Mould is present in bakery goods long before it becomes visible and, together with yeast, still contributes to the aetiology of many ailments that humans have suffered from since urbanisation.

Moulds and yeast, if eaten beyond the capacity of our immune system, can cause what is termed dysbiosis. This is a state in which the normal bowel flora has been changed to predominantly unhealthy organisms. A host of problems is associated with dysbiosis ranging from any type of digestive complaint to immune system weaknesses.[52] Candidiasis[53] (caused by an overgrowth of a yeast organism) is one such condition involving dysbiosis, and an anti-Candida regime usually includes the reduction of exposure to yeast and mould from dietary sources.

Urban settler would have been exposed to an extraordinary amount of dietary yeasts and moulds not only due to the consumption of bread and other bakery goods, but also because beer drinking, although fashionable before, now really began on a grand scale. Beginning with the ancient Egyptians and carrying on till very recently, a mug of beer was considered nourishment and was a normal part of the diet for many people. Nowadays, some people still believe that beer has health giving properties and they usually quote the vitamin B content of beer as the reason for this. But beer encourages large-scale yeast overgrowth and is therefore not a healthy type of alcoholic drink. It also leaves an acidic ash in the human body, contributing to a poor acid-alkaline balance as explained above. And many middle and lower class urban settlers ate meals that consisted of mainly bread and beer; a feast for moulds and yeasts in their guts.

In urban settlements, mould was not only present in foods, but it also reached urban settler through the general atmosphere. Building houses of stone brought with it insufficient circulation of fresh air. This in turn encouraged a

---

52 Hooper LV, Gordon JI. Commensal host-bacterial relationships in the gut. Science. 2001; 292: 1115-1

53 Kane JG, Chretien JH, and Garagusi VE. Diarrhoea caused by Candida. Lancet. 1976; (7955): 335-36

degree of house dust to collect and mould to grow, neither of which was ever completely absent. Condensation on the inside of stone walls encouraged the growth of mould, and vacuum cleaners were not yet invented to suck up human skin residues, dirt particles and little creatures feeding on these. Urban dweller was therefore exposed to a critical mass of mould and dust that may well have tipped the scales in favour of these hazards becoming a permanent irritant.[54]

By now, we may have an inkling which miasm is associated with early urbanisation. Yeasts and moulds, poor waste elimination, weight and fat gain as well as a general disinclination to physical activity all point at... Sycosis!

The story continues.

Refined Grains, Blood Sugar and the Adrenal Glands

By about 500 BC the Romans established a milling system by which five grades of flour could be produced. The finest was reserved for the upper classes as it produced the much desired white loaf. However, the Romans realised this was void of nutrition and their gladiators were given coarse grain bread to keep them well-nourished and strong.

Although the refining of grains happened late in the story of urbanisation, it nevertheless caused a further reduction of nutrients from the diet of upper class citizens, who already suffered from poor living habits.

Additionally, it strained the blood sugar balancing mechanisms. (Refined flour is digested and its sugars released into the blood very quickly. Insulin secretion therefore has

---

54 Gray MR, et al. Mixed mould mycotoxicosis: immunological changes in humans following exposure in water-damaged buildings. Arch. Environmental Health. 2003 Jul; 58(7):410-20

to surge beyond what humans are designed to handle in the long run.) This brought with it functional disturbances of blood sugar balance including adrenal insufficiency. It also caused a new kind of stress – an endogenous stress response entirely induced by the release of adrenaline, growth hormone and cortisol during low blood sugar episodes. These hormones accompany the process of bringing blood sugar back up to normal before the next meal is consumed. This is a vital mechanism that protected humans from collapse during periods of poor food supply. But it was not meant to be set in motion three times per day and on a more extreme scale. (The more insulin is secreted, the lower the blood sugar falls and therefore the more adrenalin, growth hormone and cortisol are released.)

As we said, the stress response is designed to be an emergency mechanism for flight and fight or for times of poor nutrition. Our bodies can handle it well. However, if abused by wrong nutrition and poor life-style choices as seen during urbanisation and maintained to this day, it produces a gradual decline of adrenal function. It also causes a gradual decline of any other mechanism of the body that is linked to stress hormones. We may think of the heart which responds to adrenaline, or the thyroid gland.

It is most interesting that low adrenal output has an adverse effect on the conversion of thyroid hormones to their active state and on the transport of thyroid hormones into cells. Adrenal stress therefore may have reduced the already sluggish thyroid activity and lowered metabolic rate of the Psoric individual to even lower levels.

In addition, just as with nomad but in augmented fashion, poor cortisol output would have lead to an increase in allergic tendencies, now probably directed towards a critical mass of dust and mould. All very Sycotic.

But the really worrying consequences are found in the increased secretion of growth hormone during the stress response. This may well be the physiological proof of our Sycotic tendency to growths and it may even be the basis for cancer once Sycosis is suppressed. Growth hormone acts via its mediator IGF-1 which is being investigated for its carcinogenic capacity because it causes hyperproliferation as well as reduction of programmed cell death.[55] An excess of growth hormone also causes oedema or water-logging of tissues, again a Sycotic trait.

But humans are resilient. In early urban days the effect from growth hormone and other stress hormones would be primarily functional, because however ill-balanced and mouldy the diet was, it still consisted of foods free of artificial chemicals. Also, pollution from other sources was minimal and the human body was therefore not under the sort of strain that it is now.

Sugar

The whole problem of strain on the adrenal glands was compounded once sugar or other sweeteners were abused on a grand scale, probably from about 500 BC onwards. Sugar does not only damage the blood sugar balancing mechanisms, it also reduces the activity of immune cells for several hours after ingestion. In addition, sugar digestion and assimilation uses up valuable nutrients such as the vitamin B complex without filling up body stores with

---

55 Platz, EA, et al. Plasma insulin-like growth factor 1and binding protein -3 and subsequent risk of prostate cancer in the PSE era. Cancer Causes Control.2005; 16:255-62

anything but pure monosaccharide. The vitamins of the B family have many functions in our body, but one most important one is to help the conversion of glucose to energy. So eating glucose but reducing vitamin B stores at the same time is not a good idea.

People who eat a lot of sugar therefore are at risk of developing poor energy, blood sugar problems and poor resistance to infection.

Diet across the Classes

For a long time it was mostly the upper classes that could afford to drown their sorrows in sugar and refined flour. The rest only indulged occasionally, or not at all. The saving grace of the upper classes was probably the fact that they could also afford to eat a lot of meat. This helped their much abused adrenal glands because protein eaten at the same time as carbohydrate reduces the insulin curve to less extreme. On the other hand, fresh vegetables and fruit probably became less fashionable as they were seen as less expensive and so less desirable.

The less privileged ate coarser grains and less sugar, but also less meat and probably also not many fresh vegetables and fruit. This is because transport and storage became an issue, with fresh produce going off quickly in the hot climate of Mesopotamia and the Mediterranean. Animals, on the other hand, could be driven into town alive and slaughtered locally, their meat purchased and cooked on a daily basis.

Grains could be stored for many months and so probably were the staple of the middle and lower classes.

On the whole, each class had advantages as well as disadvantages to their diet, so that the general health of every class suffered equally. However, it is significant for our discussion of miasms to note that the upper classes and to some degree the more affluent members of the middle classes became prone to a new type of metabolic dysfunction to do with adrenal insufficiency.

Sycotic Behaviour, or the Urban Female

In a way one feels sorry for the early-day noble and affluent female. With nothing to do in the morning, continuing with a rather quiet afternoon, finishing off with a free evening, she really had a life of leisure stretching ahead into the endless future of nothingness. But remembering where she came from, we know that she had a make-up that was originally hunter-gatherer, then agricultural or nomadic. How could such a female survive the void?

Let us remember how she did it before, as Psoric or Tubercular woman – she was busy with her chores, complaining all the way, but at least doing something with a purpose. When frustrated she drowned it in cereal carbs (opiate cycle) or alcohol, or engaged in physical activity appropriate for a nomadic woman (dancing, gossiping or arguing). On the whole she was OK, just functioning under par, with some chronic skin issues, diarrhoea, constipation or acute respiratory complaints hitting her more often than not.

Now a woman of noble birth or affluent circumstance, she felt physically sluggish, puffy (oedema) and strangely fatigued without having done much at all. This was way beyond periodical boredom. This was unbearable 24-7 on all levels and it had to be remedied as otherwise she would have descended into madness (which some did anyway).

Available for this purpose were newly emerging entertainments in the way of retail therapy, beauty therapy, abusing

91

stimulants as physical pick-me-ups, bullying servants and a bit of cruelty on holidays when a seat at the Circus Maximus would guarantee spectacles involving live humans being eaten by even more alive animals.

Drawn-out dinner parties featuring ever more exotic dishes (more stimulation) led to orgies where overeating became fashionable. Beautiful slave girls dancing accompanied by gorgeous slave men playing musical instruments and reciting poetry all observed by bored noblemen and women inebriated by too much food and drink. One thing led to another…

Urban man and woman discovered sex as entertainment. Never before was it seen as a way to spend otherwise idle time, but now – eureka! – the penny dropped.

I suppose that various sexual deviancies emerged round about the same time and served the same purpose.

Now was also the time for prostitution. There was no hiding in a small settlement or in a clan, but early cities provided a degree of anonymity. The underprivileged female soon found that however much a noble man despised her in principle, in practice he did not. In this way, prostitution emerged as a new phenomenon and served to mix genetic material between poor and rich as well as spread acute infections of the venereal and non-venereal kind.

Going back to our urban female, her menses developed into a disastrous affair, with irregularities and accompanied by much bleeding and pain. The tubercular tendency to inflammation now spread to the reproductive and genital areas. Why this shift took place can be explained in several ways.

First, adrenal insufficiency is associated with thyroid problems as well as oestrogen, progesterone and testosterone imbalances. In this way, the wealthy urban female increasingly suffered from reproductive hormone imbalances.

Secondly, her newly found sexual liberation invited all sorts of acute venereal infections which revelled in the soil of poor nutrition, weakened immunity and a critical mass of moulds and yeasts all preparing the environment for gonorrhoea, chlamydia, syphilis et al.

Please note that these infectious organisms, just as scabies and tuberculosis, had been around for a long time and probably had caused minor acute problems now and again, which humans had been able to shake off without any drama. But in the urban female and male (he was subject to the same behaviours and circumstances as the female) conditions were right for the problem to get out of hand. Even so, it is unreasonable to suggest that an acute gonorrhoea infection can cause chronic asthma or arthritis in the next generation. There has to be more to it.

Sycotic Attitude Married to Sycotic Stimulus

As it was with Psora and Tuberculosis, Sycosis was caused by a general attitude married to specific behaviour patterns. This combination was sustained over many generations by a critical mass of people. The attitude of class society was seen as advantageous by many, otherwise it would not have been sustained. The alternative was worse and that is why many humans moved out of their Psoric and/or Tubercular mentality. In turn, the Sycotic behaviour that was adapted by urban dweller was an answer to the new problems of class society as described above.

Both together matched perfectly as one arose out of the other in logical manner. They also matched in depth or severity as the anxiety about fitting in, sustaining status or rising up in society was deeper than the basic survival anxiety of Psora. If urban dweller did not fit in, he was ostracised. Life had become anonymous, and clan and family ties had dissolved in a way that putting a foot wrong could leave you trampled on and isolated forever. This kind of worry was new to urban dweller. In Psoric and Tubercular times blood ties were sacrilegious. But now, your family could easily turn on you just to save their own skin. For a homeopath it may be interesting to learn that an irreversible split or break in family ties can cause adrenal fatigue. It may therefore be possible that the threat of losing one's place and security within society caused a continuous and gradual worsening of adrenal function (reinforced by the other behaviours and factors discussed above).

The message for homeopaths is that we do not need gonorrhoea to explain Sycosis. In fact we cannot achieve a cure if we think that there was no Sycosis before gonorrhoea because we will ignore other factors which continuously maintain Sycosis.

The problem is that our anti-sycotic remedies are arrived at with the idea of gonorrhoea in mind. Taking away gonorrhoea, will they still cure Sycosis? To some extent, yes. But we also need to remove all Sycotic maintaining causes that we have identified above. And probably there are more that we have not recognised yet.

Urban Stress and Spirituality

On the whole, urban life was stressful also from an emotional point of view. The stress of maintaining one's livelihood was now full on again, having been temporarily relieved by Psora and Tuberculosis.

Now, however, stress was not caused by immediate and acute survival anxiety as during hunter-gatherer times and also not by chronic background anxiety about grain stores, weather conditions and hostile clans. It was caused by a host of emotions associated with class war.

More often than not decisions had to be made according to what other people would think and how they would rate you. Arrogance and despicable behaviour towards the socially lower individual became common practice. Kicking lower-class youngsters, spitting on them, pushing them in the dirt, making them walk in the gutter etc – arrogant attitudes that served to establish in the victim feelings of self-disgust early on in life, when a person has no inner understanding or self-defence by intellectual means. These feelings became ingrained as a person grew up and brought with them a continuous stream of negative emotional self-image, anxiety and social acceptance issues that – as we know today – had (and still have) tremendous adverse effects on the immune-endocrine–nervous system axis.[56] Never before did homo sapiens cause himself so much suffering purely by losing his self-belief and by worrying continuously how he would look to the Joneses.

And as there is always someone better off or higher up in the ranking, everyone was affected to some degree, even the noble individual. However, in such a person, concern about his standing in society would be expressed as arrogance, as in our homeopathic Platina personality.

---

56 Kandel E. A new intellectual framework for psychiatry. Am J Psychiatry. 1998; 155:457-69

Ray O. How the mind heals and hurts the body. Am Psychol. 2004; 59(1):29-40

Further, worries about fitting in and being OK on the surface caused urban man to on the one hand go out and try harder to be acceptable and on the other hand feel isolated and alone in his anxiety which he could never admit to.

There was no natural or healthy relief for any of these new aspects to human emotions. As we know exercise gives us endorphins, but urban man did not get much of this. Daylight and sunshine makes us happy, but urban man had learnt to shun this, as dark skin became a tell-tale sign of the working man. The diet was getting more and more devoid of fresh food and so void of vitality, thereby further reducing man's positive energy. Spending time in nature itself – as some people believe – could have helped some to find their inner peace, but this was not in vogue anymore. We can see how urban life brought with it emotional instability and anxiety but no way to soothe it.

Spirituality was of course man's only hope and many urban people rediscovered this area afresh and with renewed vigour. At least there were some Gods who – if one obeyed their wishes – would still accept even the most lowly, dirty and disgusting individual (as this is how some began thinking of themselves).

We mentioned under Psora and Tuberculosis that man, since the light bulb went on, had been practising dualistic spirituality. Hunter-gatherer would have subscribed to a kind of animism, where every tree and river would hold a spirit. This made sense since hunter-gatherer lived in nature and depended completely on other organisms and features which shared his environment, i.e. the tree bearing fruit, the river for fish and fresh water.

Psoric man became more specific and began attributing every important job or area in his life to a particular god, thereby inventing gods for harvest, rain, sunshine, but also fertility and good fortune. Psoric spirituality therefore reflected the social evolutionary stage man was at.

Tubercular spirituality was similar to Psoric but with more emphasis on seasons, good fortune, fertility, guidance, protection of the herd, and so forth.

Now that man had entered the urban phase of social evolution, the gods not only had to become better educated and step up their expertise, they also began fighting amongst themselves predominantly for rank and power.

The first urban civilisations began inventing a network of gods, each responsible for very specific jobs. By the time the Greeks and Romans had their say, the gods had taken on a mind of their own. Infighting, intrigue, cruelty, incest and cunning on Olympus reflected human life down on earth. Humans did not have much to do with the gods, except when they were unfortunate enough to be subject of their wrath or of some out of proportion act of revenge or punishment.

The idea of the benevolent god who forgave sins as long as you repented did not arrive till Jesus spread this concept. Till then, your punishment might have been reduced in severity, but punished you would be – even if you repented. Tribulations that hit urban dweller – such as perhaps loss of business, illness or death of a child – were often interpreted as punishments for spiritual or other crimes committed.

And since there were so many different gods it was hard to appease them all, and one was bound to make a mistake at some point.

Thus, the mentality and excess of urban life was reflected in the mentality of the gods and the excesses of heaven. Not only was there excess in the number of gods but also in the acts they committed and the behaviour they exhibited.

Some lucky urban dwellers may have found their peace in spirituality; but on the whole, spirituality probably only reinforced their problems without offering any solutions. The general unaccountability of the Sycotic gods did nothing to put an anxious mind to rest; quite the opposite.

The more confident person, as always, moved about unperturbed, seeking out advantage and gain at every opportunity and triumphing over his less fortunate and emotionally volatile peer.

But apart from advantages for the individual, why did Sycosis spread and take hold over millennia to come?

Benefits of Sycosis

We said that humans moved into Sycosis because they perceived the need to become even less dependent on nature. Further division of labour allowed this to happen (for some). Thus a society developed where status and wealth became more, and physical labour and strength less, desirable. The downsides of this development have been discussed above.

But were there any upsides that allowed Sycosis to remain in vogue for millennia to this day? We know by now that only a collectively perceived advantage would have allowed a miasm to take hold and spread.

Yes, there were considerable advantages for many people. First of all, the more affluent members of society were obviously better off than before. There was no way that an urban dweller of respectable status such as a lawyer or secretary would go back to ploughing fields or milking cows. A bit of chaos could be endured as a price, and there was always hope that he or his children would rise up even higher on the social ladder.

But beyond personal gain, on a collective scale Sycosis allowed for physical, emotional and mental liberation and emancipation to take place. The seed of adventure and courage contained in the Tubercular spirit now found fertile soil in the Sycotic need to expand and go beyond the previously possible. The mind went where it had never gone before. The body followed. Many mistakes were made, but this is how we learnt. Had we not tried, we would have stayed stuck in the muddy waters of Psora and the bogs of Tuberculosis.

In this way much academic achievement is down to Sycosis, as the Sycotic mind collects facts, information and knowledge just as greedily as the body craves fats, spices and dainties. Philosophy, art, music and literature emerged and expanded our thinking and emotions. Cultural bounds were attacked and taboos were broken, paving the way to emancipation of body and mind. Without Sycosis, the age of enlightenment, emancipation of the female and the PILL would have never come about.

Whenever you find yourself holding onto limiting beliefs you need to invoke Sycosis to break down your chains. Go where you have not dared to tread and do it with Sycotic exuberance. Remember, a bit of Sycosis is still better than Cancer, so let go and go wild once in a while.

Which brings us to....

Recreational Drugs

Mind-altering substances derived from plants had arrived on the middle-eastern and European stage by 4000 BC. Sumerians, Assyrians, Minoans, Egyptians and later Greeks and Romans used these extensively. Evidence was found even in neolithic graves in Switzerland. The opium poppy and cannabis were the plants cultivated for this purpose.

It is thought that cannabis was employed by priests to achieve a state of enlightenment, much as a large variety of mind-altering substances have been used throughout the world and by all cultures through the ages. But opium, thanks to its anaesthetic properties, was employed by priests for more sinister purposes. It allowed priests to perform acts of "magic", however illusory, in order to manipulate their congregation. This gives us a first clue as to which path our miasmatic train will take from now on.

Opium, with its tremendous pain relieving properties, was also treasured by ancient surgeons; in Egypt, ancient documents were found describing its use even for teething pains of babies. By Victorian times, laudanum (an opium preparation) was used by a large proportion of the British and probably European population. Its use was so wide-spread that most children would have been introduced to it whilst still breastfeeding to prevent colic and teething pain, thus heralding in the age of paracetamol.

In the second century AD, the roman emperor Severus released Opium for use by the general public and it became available for purchase on common street markets.

A mind-altering drug of this class must have left its mark. Whilst we are well aware of its addictive qualities and of the physiological effects of long-term use, have we ever stopped and considered what traces it left on our collective mental/emotional attitude?

One important clue is found in the use of opium by soldiers. Since early Mesopotamian times, opium was treasured by war-lords and soldiers alike. Its special properties numbed the soldier to the terrors ahead and so made him more courageous and battle-ready. Once injured, opium relived pain and kept soldiers going.

How did Alexander and his men conquer most of the "known" world? How did the Roman Empire expand? Was it only due to superior organisation, tactics and resources, or did they get a little extra help?

To leave no doubt in your mind at all about opiate and other drug use by military commanders, the following is an extract from an article in the German magazine Der Spiegel by A. Ulrich, 6th May 2005:

"Many of the Wehrmacht's soldiers were high on Pervitin (Speed) when they went into battle, especially against Poland and France – in a Blitzkrieg fuelled by speed. The German military was supplied with millions of methamphetamine tablets during the first half of 1940. The drugs were part of a plan to help pilots, sailors and infantry troops become capable of superhuman performance. The military leadership liberally dispensed such stimulants, but also alcohol and opiates, as long as it believed drugging and intoxicating troops could help it achieve victory over the Allies. But the Nazis were less than diligent in monitoring side-effects like drug addiction and a decline in moral standards."

What sort of decline we are talking about, we are well aware of. I assume that the higher ranks and even the command structures were also high most of the time and this includes concentration camp commanders and staff.

While opium and other drugs were widely used, the monumental significance this had for humanity on a collective scale needs to be discussed just a little more in detail.

Opium is a superb anaesthetic. This enabled man to develop a certain blasé attitude towards pain. Opium also has a general numbing effect on all emotions. The sum total of both of these attributes produced a significant shift in attitude. Man was becoming less concerned about the physical and emotional pain his fellow was experiencing. In other words, empathy and sympathy gradually became some of the less common human traits. One could go as far as suspecting a complete absence of emotions in many individuals who used opium on a regular basis.

And if you do not feel pain and cannot feel empathy with someone else's, and if you have a miasmatic tendency to being bored and aggressive, you may begin losing your inhibitions to being actively cruel. Perhaps to stir up some last remnant of physical sensation you have left in you.

Going back to our priests (Babylonian, Assyrian, Egyptian, Roman), drug use turned out to be a major player on the miasmatic stage. It allowed priests to claim back some of the power they lost during urbanisation.

As clan mages they had had significant might, but amongst city dwellers the mind had begun to liberate itself. The anonymity of city life allowed some less naïve individuals to hide their scepticism and get by unnoticed. Also, money and possessions were now found to be of more direct importance and influence on one's fortune and well-being than the gods, so that spirituality and its officials lost some of its influence. The poor man experienced such an amount of injustice and lack of charity that his faith began to wane too. He may have begun challenging the natural order of things and this posed a threat to the upper classes.

By and by, priests tried to regain their power by using opium during staged acts of miraculous healing and pain-less injuries etc. This continuously re-established and maintained the ties of dependency between the simple man and religious officials. Secular rulers were well aware of the hoax but it served their purpose too. The masses had to remain submissive. And what better means than using mental and emotional control. It helped that in urban society, priests were often from noble families, keeping both branches of power in the hands of the rich and wealthy.

Since drug use was widespread amongst urban populations, priests and noblemen of influence also used drugs for their own entertainment. It fed the Sycotic spirit of needing stimulation and excitement and became part of daily life.

Nowadays we are well aware of the consequences of long-term drug use. Mental imbalances and mental disease are common effects, but heart, respiratory and liver disease are also found on a regular basis.

In particular, paranoia and problems with perception of reality are very prominent, and when present to a subtle degree go by almost unnoticed by the victim and his sur-roundings. Any slightly odd behaviour will be put down to personality and not drug use.

I believe that the use of drugs introduced a slightly differ-ent flavour to our Sycotic attitude which until now was basically concerned with status and entertainment. Drugs introduced numbing of sympathy and readiness to commit cruelty beyond reason. Thus the chaos did not remain innocent but took a decidedly evil turn.

This state could not be sustained indefinitely. Man began suffering again and thus the search for a solution was on once more. What better way to contain chaos and cruelty than by imposing order?

And so humanity hailed in the rise of discipline, but left Syphilis in its wake. How did this next miasm come about?

Monotheism

To a great degree, it was monotheism which sorted out the chaos in the Western world.

As discussed above, the endless turmoil within Middle Eastern and Mediterranean polytheism did nothing to calm the Sycotic mind. In fact, it produced ever more anxiety as the Gods were cruel and unaccountable. There was no way of knowing how to escape their wrath and lead a quiet life.

Monotheism, on the other hand, introduced the idea of one God, who was almighty and asked strict adherence to a clear set of rules. These rules were simple and easy to follow, at least on the surface, so that life for the believer in one God became structured and initially quite peaceful compared to the chaos that reigned beforehand. Rites of washing, fasting, birth, death and marriage were introduced and the one God appeared decidedly benevolent and accountable, at least for those who decided to follow and obey him. Life became simpler, more secure and definitely more peaceful. As social interactions became less arbitrary and more regulated, anxiety gradually subsided and a kind of faith and trust in the future took over.[57]

Pioneers of this kind of religion were again people in the Middle East.

Inspired and disciplined by Yahweh, the Israelites triumphed over chaotic and undisciplined neighbouring tribes and established themselves as one of the fitter societies in the Middle East and Europe. (And fittingly, the name

[57] The peace conveyed by monotheism was nevertheless continuously interrupted either by people who did not adhere to it, or those who only paid lip-service to it. In this way monotheism only brought with it the option of peace.

"Israel" means, roughly translated 'one who struggled with God and found himself'). To this day, historians quote the well structured and disciplined way of life and the strict and enlightened hygienic rules amongst Jewish populations of European cities as the reason for high survival rates during plagues and other epidemics. There was a definitive advantage to be found in strict discipline and communal support amongst close-knit religious communities.

Although Yahweh was at times unforgiving if his rules were not obeyed, this trait was probably necessary in order to discipline the citizens of proverbial Sodom and Gomorrah.

Interestingly, the Sycotic mind only responds to threats and physical aggression as disciplinary measures. Reasoning, star charts and rewards are completely lost on the Sycotic child and will never achieve anything. In this way, the mentality of the God Yahweh reflected once more the mentality of the people who invented him. However, Yahweh kept his children in check and so discipline and order was established and maintained for considerable periods of time.

By the time Jesus came along, the "known" world was firmly in the hand of the Romans. Resistance against Rome was fruitless and so the God who emerged was necessarily peaceful. (Unfortunately the Church would stray far from this path in the millennia to come). Recognising that resistance to Rome would have meant annihilation, Jesus encouraged inner peace and feelings of love and charity to promote some degree of happiness in this life. As a reward he promised eternal life to the reformed and no punishment for anyone, reformed or not. These principles gave "enslaved societies" a way to transcend their prover-bial yoke, a peaceful way to live in slavery without being unhappy. Thus was set the scene for Cancer, the miasm. But it took two millennia for Cancer to take hold and much happened meanwhile.

In 600 BC, Muhammad rose. His advent was overdue and most welcome. Since the destruction of the Roman Empire, the Middle East had descended into worse chaos than ever. In towns, opium, cannabis and alcohol consumption was high and as a consequence morals, routines and personal discipline were almost non-existent. Townspeople were subject to arbitrary rules and rulers and to raids by nomad tribes who were a law unto themselves.

Muhammad sorted this out to a great degree. He most significantly protected females and their offspring by ensur-ing their safety within an Islamic marriage. (If you think that nowadays an Islamic marriage is a poor fate for many women, please be aware that the alternative at the time of Muhammad was infinitely worse, as most females had no legal protector and relied entirely on male charity and mercy which, needless to say, often did not materialise.) Muhammad also brought in a strict set of routines to dis-cipline any excess. Prayers many times per day and fasting rituals brought in the unruly and helped them to lead a constructive life. No doubt, the Middle East was better off with Islam than before Islam.

Again, Islam reflects the need to discipline by force as so many followers were, and still are, predominantly Sycotic. This is perhaps why we still see harsh physical punishments in some Islamic countries. Regrettable it is; but from a homeopathic point of view it makes sense.

Today just about 50% of the world population are monotheistic or live in monotheistic societies even if they themselves do not practice monotheism. Monotheistic mentality, and we will discuss what exactly I mean by this, therefore shapes about 50% of the world's population. How this is linked to Syphilis we will discuss later.

The East did not acquire monotheism but still produced the Syphilitic miasm. Have we finally found a flaw in our theory?

No, we have not, because in East Asia at least, discipline was promoted not through monotheism but by the philosophy of one of the most influential human beings that ever walked the planet. This man, who lived about 500 BC in China, helped shape the mentality of the East and with it the mentality of at least 2 billion people today. Who am I taking about? It is of course Confucius.[58]

Confucianism

Confucius was Chinese and his and his followers' teachings strongly influence to this day most of East Asia, but particularly China, Japan, Korea, Taiwan, Vietnam and other areas where Chinese people settled. Much as monotheistic mentality tints about 50% of the world's population even if not necessarily every person is a practising monotheist, most of East Asia – and that would be about 2 billion people living in the area bordered by Mongolia in the north, the Philippines in the East, Indonesia in the South and China

58 India is affected by the Syphilitic miasm partially through monotheistic Islam, as about 13.5% of the Indian population are Muslim. Even if Hindus were not affected, this would be a significant proportion of the population. But Hinduism also has some Syphilitic aspects. The rigid class system as well as the idea of karma and reincarnation as tools for reward and punishment play their part in the genesis of Syphilis. On the whole, though, Hindusim is not Syphilitic, as the concept of heresy is absent and liberal thinking, charity and tolerance prevail.

in the West – interpret the world in a Confucian way. That's about 33% of the world's population.

And Confucius' influence did not stop in Asia. Jesuit translations were brought back to Europe by missionaries in the 17th century where thinkers of the Age of Enlightenment built some Confucian ideas into Renaissance philosophy, especially those on morality.

Confucianism is based on the idea that man can improve himself through self-cultivation. In particular one should cultivate virtue and strive to develop moral perfection.

Two cardinal values permeate all Confucian thought and these are humanism and ritual. Humanism states that all actions and thoughts should be based on goodness, compassion and kind-heartedness. This applies to all people including leaders, making Confucianism politically important.

Ritual, the other cardinal value, refers to the propriety of everyday behaviour. It is not meant to describe harsh religious or self-disciplinary measures, but is supposed to help shape everyday life to promote health and contentedness. One could for instance mention regular bed times, daily exercise and healthy food choices as part of this cardinal value.

One important aspect of Confucianism was the introduction of meritocracy which created an alternative to the nobility of blood by accepting nobility of virtue and education. Confucius proclaimed that through self-education any person could better his position in society, and this idea became mainstream practice in Confucian China (although nobility of blood was never abolished until communism took hold). Through passing the Imperial examination system, for instance, anyone could become a government official, thereby bettering his and his family's standing and wealth considerably.

At the time these ideas were revolutionary – up to this point Eastern society had progressed along the same lines as the West, with urbanisation leading to class war, excess and cruelty. We can recognise in hindsight that Confucius and his followers bestowed Eastern Sycotic societies with order and peace and enabled the East to move forward instead of drown in its own chaos. By promoting self-discipline, routine, moral values, humaneness and education, Confucianism went straight to the heart of the Sycotic matter as Sycosis promoted lack of boundaries, chaos, excess, selfishness, moral decline, cruelty and one-upmanship. Status and social climbing was vitally important, but mostly achieved by cheating, bribing and intrigue. Confucianism changed all this without weapons or force. I believe the time was right; a critical mass of people had suffered enough and needed to find a solution. Confucius offered the only solution possible, i.e. an active attempt at self-improvement and discipline of the individual and a change of attitude on a collective scale. Humanity in the East needed to move on or be doomed; it was simply a matter of collective survival.

Interestingly, Confucian ideas as described above have become such an integral part of our present day attitude in East and West that we hardly recognise it as anything foreign or unusual. It seems that Confucianism somehow just expresses common sense or, even more, something somehow intrinsic in human nature – but actually it took humanity many millennia to reach this state.

For our miasmatic discussion, all we need to remember at this point is that the East overcame Sycosis and chaos with the help of Confucianism, the West by employing monotheism. Both achieved the same state of collective discipline, surely an advantage after Sycotic excess and chaos.[59]

Sycosis and Syphilis – Two Sides of the Same Coin

As homeopaths we often see Sycosis and Syphilis as two sides of the same coin. Our main remedies for one often cover the other almost to the same degree, examples being Thuja, Nitric Acid and Mercury. Alternatively, we find that having treated Sycosis, suddenly Syphilis rears its ugly head with a vengeance – and vice versa. No other two miasms are so closely related. But our conventional descriptions of excess for Sycosis and destruction for Syphilis do nothing to explain this phenomenon.

Through our new perspective we now get a viable explanation. Syphilis helps to discipline Sycotic traits. And Sycosis helps to liberate us from Syphilitic chains. We need both, but in balance!

What then is the connection between monotheism, discipline and Syphilis?

Discipline

Discipline is the art of self-containment in the promotion of self-advancement. This is my definition and shall be the

---

59 The progression of miasm from pre-Psoric through Psora/Tuberculosis to Sycosis and Syphilis did not mean that all individual human beings progressed. In fact some remained behind and so all miasmatic attitudes and states exist simultaneously to this day. What did progress was human society on a collective scale so that new miasms came into being. And whilst society solved its problems and moved on, chronic disease got worse and caused physical decline on a collective scale.

one referred to here. It expresses the idea that in order to get on in life, even if this just means staying alive and not promoting one's own premature death, we need to learn to curtail all unhelpful impulses and at the same time judiciously augment and employ all helpful ones. Discipline in the first instance has nothing to do with punishment, self-chastisement, denial or ascetics.

Most human beings acquire discipline naturally by trial and error, simply by learning that some things are not helpful and others are. We even have the capacity to learn degrees and variations of discipline in this way, meaning we can learn that some behaviours are fine up to a threshold or in certain situations, but not in others or not above a certain threshold.

I believe that this kind of acquired discipline is intrinsic in human nature and it serves our survival as an individual and species.

However, there was a (Sycotic) time in our social history when we lost this natural ability. Perhaps the reason was that we found ourselves in a situation (urbanisation) that we had not been in before and that promoted a lack of discipline. Before we could learn enough about this situation, it had already got out of hand on a collective scale and stayed out of hand to this day on some level. Natural – let us call it instinctual or pre-programmed discipline – could not contain the forces of Sycosis. It would need more than that.

Having said this, history tells us that almost as soon as Sycosis became rampant, the antidote sprang to life. It is as if the problem itself already contained the solution. Monotheism as a disciplinary measure (practised first by ancient Hebrew tribes) arrived on the scene somewhere around 1900 BC, so about 2000 years after urbanisation began. (Actually, there was also a short period of monotheism practiced in ancient Egypt around 1300 BC, but it was abolished very soon.)

The discipline of monotheism, as we already discussed, attempted to overcome Sycosis by using the power of the mind, as our natural intrinsic discipline was too weak when faced with Sycotic excess. This made the three main monotheistic religions quite cerebral in their approach. As we know, a substantial amount of schooling is required to become an adult member of a congregation. The training can involve memorizing of script, formal prayers and rituals and the process can take many months. Interestingly, this usually takes place just before puberty begins, at a time when a person would naturally awake to their bodily urges. In our discussion of miasms, we recognise at this point how much the body is denied (as the body wants to be Sycotic) while the mind is employed to overcome physical impulses. Many tasks that keep the mind occupied such as reciting verses, prayers and psalms are used tactically as diversions from bodily needs and desires. The power and capacity of the mind is augmented and the body is neglected. Routines such as prayer times, washing and fasting as well as time spent in congregation all serve the purpose of regulating daily life and providing a framework from which people can operate constructively. Religious laws pertaining to social life and contracts between people helped to establish simple and clear guidelines and this helped reduce bribery, cheating and intrigue. People felt empowered and began breathing easier. There was hope after all.

The whole monotheistic air castle was built on, and enforced by, the idea that God knows and sees all. Heavenly threats and rewards were enough to keep people in check who were used to unpredictable, revengeful and bloodthirsty gods. But the most powerful factor which kept the whole thing going was that it worked. Monotheism brought peace and order back to whole communities, or at least to significantly large sectors of communities. It was a definite advantage and nobody in their wildest dreams would have turned back.

For our discussion of miasms, it has become clear that the attitude which posed as susceptibility for Syphilis was the need to overcome chaos (Sycosis) with the help of discipline. Society was in desperate need to contain its excesses on all levels and the measure of discipline provided by monotheism and Confucianism did just that.

So what went wrong? Why did chronic disease get worse especially in those individuals and sectors of society which managed to discipline themselves?

Perversion

Of course, many factors came together to move disease onto deeper levels. As always, the mind, or rather the prevailing attitude (our susceptibility) played an important part.

As discussed above, natural mechanisms of containing chaos and excess had long been lost, overpowered by unnatural factors that had led to previous miasms. Instinct was deeply buried. What humanity was left with was the power of the mind. Human beings, however, still had a body and this body had demands.

Before full-blown syphilis developed on all levels, only the mind was affected, giving us our susceptibility. As the mind tried to discipline the body, this body was still Sycotic. The mind moving towards Syphilis therefore had a major problem. The Sycotic body-beast rearing its tail was difficult to slay. One managed intermittently, but it just came back with a vengeance. The mental effort required became more and more strenuous and eventually a line was crossed. Constructive discipline turned into perversion.

Lying on beds of nails, endless fasting, self-flagellation, religious masochism and ritual mutilation of genitals are such examples of Syphilitic perversion in the name of discipline. Unfortunately, this rather destructive attitude or interpretation of discipline did not stop at self-harm. Many practices became routine and were forced onto the young generation who grew up believing that this was the right thing to do, although it caused the body so much pain. Thus denial of the body deepened from generation to generation. Always finding intellectual reasons for physical crimes.

Eventually, when we reach full-blown Syphilis, we see large scale perversions on national level such as the Crusades, the Inquisition, the trans-Atlantic slave trade, annihilation of indigenous peoples, Communism, Dictatorship, Fascism and the Holocaust.

What do these very dark chapters of human history all have in common?

Large-scale and purposefully organised execution of acts of cruelty against fellow human beings. Acts so cruel that only a perverted and sick mind could have come up with them. The height of perversion, however, rests in the very fact that the perpetrators did not perceive the action as cruel, but as desired and necessary in order to keep the peace or bring well-deserved justice or prosperity to their own society.

In this way, Syphilis perverted the mind; the very mind which originally desired nothing but to contain Sycotic excesses in order to make life more peaceful and less threatening.

The Syphilitic susceptibility was the need for discipline. But what was the stimulus? What are the factors which moved the individual as well as a critical mass of people from a simple desire to control Sycosis into the most perverted realms of the mind and thus into full-blown Syphilis with its physical complaints?

We said that the mental attitude of desiring discipline deepened due to the see-saw action between mind/discipline and body/excess. But this alone would not cause Sycotic physical complaints to deepen. It is our behaviour or actions that stimulate disease and so we need to look elsewhere.

Fear and the Adrenal Glands

Our adrenal glands are one important regulator of the stress response. When we experience anxiety or fear, they kick in and secrete stress hormones. The first hormone released is adrenalin and it ensures we survive the immediate danger. Once the danger is over, we return to equilibrium. During times of stress we also secrete cortisol so that the body can sustain our self-preserving emergency measures for a longer amount of time, the time needed to for instance remove ourselves from the place of danger even further after the immediate flight has been successful. This mechanism, also called the flight or fight response, is part of our make-up and as such is a miracle of evolution.

Unfortunately it can also work to our detriment.

There are two main factors which played together to make our adrenal glands one of our weakest points. One is that the adrenals are not only turned on by mental/emotional stress, but also by low blood sugar. It is therefore any kind of stress, mental, emotional or physiological which sets in motion the adrenally mitigated stress response. Our adrenals even respond to stimulants such as coffee, tea, wine, chocolate, spices etc; all items which give us this false energy boost we know so well. When we stimulate our adrenals with caffeine etc, we literally live on borrowed time. Why this should be so brings us to the second factor – we forget again and again that our adrenal glands are part of our body and therefore need to be supplied with all the biochemical ingredients adrenal cells need in order to function. When we continuously stimulate our stress response we use up vital minerals that our adrenals need at that time as well as during periods of rest. These minerals have to come from somewhere. As we discussed before, the Psoric / Tubercular person had already started the process of depletion. After this, Sycotic man had robbed his reserves even more by indulging in stimulants and stimulating actions to keep going. Also, we must remember that Sycotic man had poor sleep patterns and therefore never gave his body the chance to carry out or complete maintenance. His adrenal glands were therefore hit by three factors: they worked too hard, they did not receive much in the way of mineral resources and also they could not regenerate damaged and destroyed cells at a satisfactory rate.

Once we arrive at Syphilis, Sycotic anxiety turns into deep-seated fear. Fear of punishment, cruelty and physical pain as described above. This type of fear affected man deeply and caused an almost continuous state of stress never experienced before. All the more so because even if a person was fortunate enough to feel relatively safe in their earthly existence (a rare occurrence!), he now was petrified of judgement day, purgatory, or whatever else he chose to believe in that would happen to him after death. He feared his afterlife because, however hard he tried, his Sycotic body would again and again entice him to sin. Syphilitic man's life was ruled by a see-sawing from extremes of pure living to perverted or otherwise sinful behaviour. Again this attitude was a question of individual perception. What was carnal sin to one was a white lie to another.

The theatrical stage that Syphilis plays on is the mind. The Syphilitic drama of eternal struggle between good and evil takes place inside the warped thoughts of its victims, completely unnoticed by the observer. The Sycotic tried to hide only his worst behaviours and only from certain people such as his wife or his employer. The Syphilitic had to hide his behaviour and actions (which were often nothing but sinful thoughts) from the entire world and even from God. A deep fear of eternal damnation gripped him and never left him, not even at night when others rested peacefully.

Nowadays, many of us have liberated ourselves from thoughts of purgatory and hell, but we remain Syphilitic to the bone. This is because we have shifted our struggle to present day issues such as health, finances and love. The present day Syphilitc will focus his fear on financial matters, on his health and looks, and on his relationships. Fear of poverty will drive a Syphilitic to extremes of stinginess or making money his only raison d'être. Fear of disease will make him germ phobic and hypochondriacal, often causing disease through the very procedures he subjects himself to in order to prevent it (multiple MRI scans, extreme diets, over-medicating himself, etc). He is focussed on his outward appearance and good looks are everything to him. This causes him to harm himself with cosmetic procedures and surgery, dieting, bulimia, over-exercising and other practices intended to improve his body image. Fear of loneliness or lack of love will cause him to enter inappropriate relationships which are either abusive or fall apart and therefore cause him to feel abandoned and lonely.

Thus the Syphilitic's life is reined by fear, although he himself does not perceive it as such. He finds the most convincing intellectual reasons for behaving the way he does, becoming a master at hiding even from himself.

Going back to our adrenal glands, once Syphilis had taken a hold and fear had become an almost permanent state of affairs, the adrenal glands could not take any more pressure, leading to chronic adrenal insufficiency of various degrees.[60] Extremes of bingeing and fasting, extremes of self-inflicted pain and extremes of nutrient deficiencies shattered adrenal reserves to near breaking point. But in order to preserve life, the body had to keep its adrenal

---

60 Bland JS, Jones D. Clinical approaches to hormonal and neuroendocrine imbalances. Functional Medicine. Chapter 32, p604ff. The Institute for Functional Medicine, 2005

Zarkovich M, Stefanova E, et al. Prolonged psychological stress suppresses cortisol secretion. Clin Endocr (Oxf).2003 Dec; 59(6);811-6

glands functioning at least to a minimum and so the pressure was taken off and moved to organs which had to this point not been affected in a major way. The law of the hierarchy of organs is how homeopaths explain this phenomenon. The more negative stimuli the body is subject to, the more organs become affected. It is as if the body, in order to preserve life, spreads the damage evenly. Better to have a number of half-working organs than two organs which do not work at all.

With the advent of Syphilis, the adrenal glands were spared from complete destruction, but thyroid, nervous system and heart became gradually compromised. The rest of the body – under the same continued pressure – shifted from poor function to destructive pathology where body parts such as enzymes, cell components and tissues progressively died. The most significant impact of this process is seen in the immune system.

Syphilis, Symmetry and the Immune System

Whereas up to this point the immune system acted to preserve the life of the individual, it now turned against it. It is as if the mental state of self-destructive practices described above is reflected in physiological processes. With regards to the immune system this meant that own body parts were now seen as the enemy. Just as the Syphilitic mind struggles to overcome Sycotic desires and forgets that those are also part of human existence, the Syphilitic immune system initiates war against other parts of the body. It thereby creates an internal physiological "civil war" against parts of the body which should actually work in tune with the very system that is trying to annihilate it. Favourite places of the immune system to attack are initially the gut (Crohn's), the skin (Psoriasis) and the thyroid gland (Hashimoto), and later more diffusely a combination of tissues as seen in Lupus. Various diseases of the nervous system (Alzheimers, Parkinsons, MS) are under investigation for being autoimmune conditions and show a further progression of Syphilis to the brain and related structures.

As we can see, Syphilis creates an unnatural state of separation on all levels. Intellect is separated from emotions as emotions are Sycotic. The mind is separated from the body as the body is Sycotic. The immune system is separated from all other body systems and begins acting as if these were a danger. In its attempt to preserve life, Syphilitic energy causes exactly that which it is trying to prevent – destruction of life. Thus we see perversion even on the physical level.

Syphilitic separation is described by Jeremy Sherr as symmetry or as being caught in a state of parallels.[61] Just as two parallel lines never meet, the Syphilitic suffers from self-imposed isolation. His mind must never give credence to his emotions; his thoughts must never consider his physiological (bodily) needs. He lives up in his head, denying and condemning anything other than intellect as animalistic and low. He talks of love, but love remains either theoretical (no true intimacy) or becomes an instrument of self-destruction (abusive relationships). Meanwhile, hidden from the rest of the world and almost hidden from himself, he is subject to an internal war taking place in his mind (moral struggle) and body (autoimmune destruction).

On a physical level the shift to auto-immune disease is mediated again, at least in part, by the lack of adrenal func-

61   Sherr J. Dynamic Materia medica, Syphilis. Dynamis Books; 2002

tion. As discussed above the adrenal hormone cortisol has many functions, one of which is to keep histamine (allergy) in check. But beyond this it also balances white blood cell activity[62] to prevent these from becoming active beyond the call of duty. When cortisol levels become chronically low as seen in adrenal fatigue of severe dimensions, white blood cells are free to savage our own body tissues.[63] This is one way for autoimmune disease to come about. It is possible that in modern day society this process has become miasmatic, i.e. that humans are already born with impaired adrenal function so that the progression to autoimmune disease is fast.

However, as always, the body is miraculously resilient. There are many types of autoimmune conditions and some are by no means life-threatening. Psoriasis, auto-immune mediated tooth decay and Vitiligo are examples of such benign conditions. Thus many people manage to live with Syphilis (the miasm) and lead a perfectly normal life.

To summarize, the attitude of needing to discipline Sycotic influences was our susceptibility to Syphilis. The stimulus that met and married with this attitude was multi-factorial and comprised of drug abuse, extreme stress invoked by witnessing or being subjected to cruelty and extreme self-disciplinary practices. More stimuli or detrimental behaviours and actions came together and I will explain these below.

---

62 Munck A, Guyre Pm, Holbrook NJ. Physiologic function of glucocorticoids in stress and their relation to pharmacologic actions. Endocr.Rev 1984; 5(1):25-44

63 Reichlin S. Neuroendocrine-immune interactions. N Eng J Med. 1993; 329(17):146-53

Fasting and the Syphilitic Diet

The Syphilitic mind believed that discipline would cure all his ills. In this he went too far.

His diet, for instance, became one of his favourite mediators of self-punishment. Religious fasting ranging in severity from excluding meat to eating nothing at all was practiced by many.

Of course there were many who simply could not afford to eat meat or any other form of quality protein on a regular basis. Syphilis took hold of these people too, as protein deficiency deepens the Sycotic condition regardless of the reasons for it.

Excluding meat without substituting it with other sources of protein (which was probably the case as people were not aware of physiological needs for protein) leads to serious problems, even when sustained for a number of days or weeks only. Protein is the building block of all cells in our body, but especially the thyroid and adrenal glands need it on a daily basis in order to replenish. The liver also needs certain building blocks of proteins (methyl and sulfyl group, cysteine, taurine, glutathione, glutamine) to keep its detoxification pathways open at all times and so a fast of one week or longer will seriously impair liver function and may even lead to liver damage. Metabolic and exogenous toxins arriving in the liver for detoxification cannot be processed without these chemical particles harvested from proteins and so remain in the liver, wreaking havoc on liver cells. Not only proteins, but also many other nutrients are needed for detoxification and most of these or their components must be supplied through diet.[64]

Now imagine a person, perhaps for religious reasons, practising harsh fasts several times per year. The liver, adrenals and thyroid will slowly but surely suffer and even longish periods between fasts do not allow recovery due to on-going dietary transgressions discussed above.

If fasting is intermittent so that only one meal is taken late in the evening or at night, this meal may disrupt our natural cortisol rhythm which normally follows our sleep-wake cycle. If we eat when we should be sleeping we may inadvertently cause an excess of cortisol to be secreted, stimulating the deposit of fat around the middle.[65] Once our cortisol rhythm has been disrupted for a period of time, it is very difficult to reset and problems with fatigue, insomnia, weight gain and infertility may ensue.

Further, overeating or eating the wrong foods after fasting causes a disruption of insulin activity. Foods high in starch such as cereal-based items as well as sugary foods raise blood sugar levels too quickly and stimulate an over-secretion of insulin which is needed to quickly shunt excess blood sugar into cells. As too much sugar is present, muscle and liver are quickly saturated and any excess is converted into fat.

If done incorrectly, therefore, fasting never leads to a tightening of the belt but quite the opposite.

(Insulin excess is also associated with insulin dependent cancers as well as insulin resistance/diabetes type 2.)

---

64 Grant D. Detoxification pathways in the liver. J Inher Met Dis. 1991;14:421-30
Lisak D, Lyon M, Jones D. Detoxification and Biotransformational Imbalances. Functional medicine. Ch22. The Institute for Functional Medicine, 2005

65 Bland JS. Clinical approaches to hormonal and neuroendocrine Imbalances. Functional medicine Ch32 p623. The Institute for Functional Medicine 2005

As the Sycotic body was already in trouble with blood sugar and adrenal balance, the Syphilitic suffered even more, depending on how harshly he treated his body.

Nowadays, whenever we see a person who sticks to severely restricted or (from our point of view) perverted dietary practices (for whatever reason) we must suspect Syphilis. Regardless of whether the diet is good or bad for him, the fact that he can stick to it at all, must mean he has sufficient discipline and therefore must be majorly Syphilitic.

Eating disorders therefore have one of their roots in Syphilis, although they probably are a combination of Sycosis (never achieving satisfaction) with Syphilis (wanting to discipline themselves and relapsing at intervals) and Cancer (desiring to achieve perfection) as we will see in the following chapters.

As homeopaths we see two interesting dietary preferences in the Syphilitic – a craving for bread and an aversion to meat. I personally believe that this can be explained by the Syphilitic desire to eat modestly and his disgust of blood and flesh, both fuelled by his inner desire to remain saintly and pure. Cancer also refuses meat, but in his case it is an ethical decision, not a physical disgust. Sycotic food preferences are all those which stimulate him. Physiologically, these foods actually have an exciting effect on his adrenal gland, giving him an artificial short term energy boost, but contributing to adrenal fatigue in the long run. Tuberculosis craves dairy which makes him sick. Psora craves starch as it calms him down and makes him able to bear the daily drudgery.

But back to Syphilis.

Do we still believe that this miasm was caused by an infection?

Syphilis

In the light of what we now understand of the Syphilitic mind-set meeting the fatigued body of the Sycotic, can we begin to see that no infection was necessary to move us into the next miasmatic picture? Was the Sycotic body not toxic and exhausted enough to need just a little more life-style abuse to turn on itself? I believe so. In the same way that gonorrhoea did not cause Sycosis and scabies did not cause Psora, syphilis did not cause Syphilis. After the body had become sufficiently weakened, the bacteria just found hospitable ground and produced the well-known disease with its four stages. Moreover, syphilis (the disease) jumped on the self-destructive train humans had already begun to board and lead them to switch to fast gear. How so?

In our defence against syphilis, we began employing mercury and later arsenic.

Mercury

The story of Syphilis is intimately linked to mercury. Mercury was used (probably from around 1000 AD onwards) to treat syphilis (the disease) and homeopaths in turn use it for the Syphilitic taint.

Interestingly, Mercury in its crude form suppresses adrenal output, especially cortisol[66]. In this way, any individual with crude mercury entering their system on a regular or even a one-off basis, will probably develop problems associ-

---

66 Gump BB, et al. Fish consumption, low-level mercury, lipids, and inflammatory markers in children. Environ Res. 2011 Oct 24; Department of Public Health, Food Studies, and Nutrition, Syracuse University, Syracuse, NY 13244, USA
Tan SW, Meiller JC, Mahaffey KR. The endocrine effects of mercury in humans and wildlife. Crit Rev Toxicol. 2009; 39(3):228-69.

ated with low cortisol levels, such as blood sugar balance, fatigue, perception of stress, sleep, allergies, chronic inflammation, cardiovascular disease and autoimmune problems.

Major sources of mercury today are seafood, dental fillings, air and water pollution, vaccinations, and exposure in utero through the mother who acquires her mercury burden in the above mentioned ways.[67]

According to a 1991 study by the W.H.O. (World Health Organization) dental fillings containing mercury release 3-17 micrograms of mercury into the bloodstream every day. The safe level established for Mercury exposure is 10 micrograms per day. It comes as no surprise that in 1997 Sweden banned mercury fillings for pregnant women, thereby giving credence to the possibility of the mercury load of a mother affecting the unborn in utero. Since then various European countries have begun phasing out mercury fillings altogether and many dentists refuse to handle mercury in their surgeries.

Proof that mercury is dangerous in very low-level exposure is found by studies examining specific immune cells targeting mercury leaching from dental fillings.[68] Another study goes even further and suggests that removal of mercury fillings improves autoimmune conditions.[69]

---

67 Holford P. New Optimum Nutirtion Bible. P 121 f. Piatkus 2004
Norouzi E, et al. Effect of teeth amalgam on mercury levels in the colostrums human milk in Lenjan. Environ Monit Assess. 2012 Jan; 184(1): 375-80
Bernhoft RA. Mercury toxicity and treatment: a review of the literature. J Environ Public Health. 2012; 460508

68 Stejskal VD, et al. Mercury-specific lymphocytes: an indication of mercury allergy in man. J Clin Immunol. 1996 Jan; 16(1):31-40.

69 Prochazkova J,et al. The beneficial effect of amalgam replacement on health in patients with autoimmunity. Neuro Endocrinol Lett. 2004 Jun; 25(3):211-8.

In short, we can assume form the general attitude towards amalgam fillings that there is something fishy about mercury and that we have not even scratched the surface of the plethora of detrimental effects this metal has on human health. Nevertheless, a start has been made in the right direction with one report. This states that mercury has been associated with damage to immune, nervous, cardiovascular, renal and dermatological systems. It affects DNA, RNA, mitochondria, enzymes and immune mechanisms.[70]

Perhaps the most firmly established link is that of mercury to autoimmune disease. Several studies show mercury exposure from amalgam fillings to be associated with autoimmunity such as thyroiditis.[71]

Recognising these effects of mercury, we can now suggest that the treatment of syphilis (the disease) with mercury would at the same time have caused deeper problems such as reduced adrenal output, inflammation, neurological damage, autoimmune disease and even psychological problems.[72] If used in the earlier stages, mercury would therefore have accelerated the progress and enforced its virulence.

In this way, mercury and syphilis may have become almost inextricably linked and produced a complex symptom picture, quite in the way that Hahnemann said medical

---

70 Hyman MH. The impact of mercury on human health and the environment. Altern Ther health med. 2004; 112(15):a862

71 Hybenova M, et al. The role of environmental factors in autoimmune thyroiditis. Neuro Endocrinol Lett. 2010; 31(3):283-9.
Suzuki Y, Inoue T, Ra C. Autoimmunity-inducing metals (hg, au and ag) modulate mast cell signaling, function and survival. Curr Pharm Des. 2011 Nov 17; (34):3805-14

72 Haynes EN, et al. Exposure to airborne metals and particulate matter and risk for youth adjudicated for criminal activity. Environ Res. 2011 Nov; 111(8):1243-8

treatments interact with the body's own disease and produce a complicated disease.

It is curious to note that, whichever way we look at it, it is not necessarily true that mercury has acted suppressively as we homeopaths like to interpret it. It may be simpler – mercury merely poisoned those treated with it. And the effects of this poisoning took a long time to show, because mercury acts hidden from view on our internal organs and mechanisms. These mechanisms being vital to our survival are extremely resilient and protected, so that any negative effects will take many years to show. This would explain why Syphilitic complaints develop unnoticed and under the surface until one day they viciously erupt and leave us almost defenceless.

If mercury was a contributing factor to moving the disease into the last stage in affected individuals, what caused the disease to become miasmatic?

The Mercury Miasm

Actually, we have already partially answered this question. In the same way that the infected mother may pass syphilis to the unborn and bring about congenital syphilis, mercury exerts its effects on the unborn, one of the two major sources of mercury poisoning for babies being exposure to it in utero (the other being vaccinations). As we have seen, a child born to a mercury poisoned mother has a high chance of being affected by mercury toxicity himself. Such a child may suffer from all the problems cited above. Also, he or she may never be able to reproduce.[73] No cause for infertility will be found as nothing is "wrong" with any

---

73 Apostoli P, Catalani S. Metal ions affecting reproduction and development. Met Ions Life Sci. 2011; 8:263-303.

organs or with the main fertility hormone producing sites such as the hypothalamus, pituitary or ovaries. "Causeless" infertility is of course another major hallmark of Syphilis.

But even if escaping infertility and still able to produce offspring, a child may be weakened and himself fall victim to disease, especially syphilis, if he lived in Syphilitic times. He would have engaged in syphilitic behaviours and triggered the disease by his actions. He may attract the bacteria and again he would be treated with mercury and so the process was perpetuated over the generations and centuries.

Ironically, neither mercury, herbs nor other compounds were effective in treating any stage of the disease and, from our point of view, just poisoned the bodies of our ancestors thereby perpetuating the problem.

Thus syphilis, the disease, was able to feed on the toxic bodies and weakened immune systems of the human species until in 1928 penicillin put a stop to it.[74]

Or did it?

Although when diagnosed, syphilis can be eradicated with penicillin, in many cases it sneakily manages to escape detection so that the tertiary stage is a common occurrence in developing countries. Diagnosed or not, syphilis is still one of our major infectious diseases today. (Curiously, nobody is working on a vaccine for syphilis, although it must be amongst the top 10 most dangerous and debilitating diseases). The WHO estimates that 12 million new cases of syphilis occur every year.[75] And syphilis increases the risk

---

74 Just before, from 1900 or so, Arsenic compounds were used, in Salvarsan, to treat syphilis. This would have increased the toxic burden of victims further.

75 WHO/TDR. The use of rabid syphilis tests. Available: http://www.who.int/ std_diagnostics/publications/manuals/Syphilis_Eng_14May07.pdf 2006; Last accessed 30th Jan 2012.

of HIV transmission by 3-5 times[76]. Co-infection with both diseases in men having sex with men occurs in 20-73% of cases.[77]

Since HIV is the ultimate autoimmune disease, we may conclude that it is the final and deepest stage of the Syphilitic miasm which does not necessarily need syphilis (the disease) to be present. Speaking of HIV, some homeopaths class it as being part of the Cancer miasm, or even being a miasm of its own.

In the Wake of Syphilis, the Miasm

Where did we go from here? We needed a miracle; there is no doubt about it. Toxic, weak and self-destructive in body and mind, the human species was doomed.

How did we survive?

For one, not everybody was affected. Some people remained behind, stuck in a relatively benign and delirious Sycotic stage. Still able to reproduce and lead a self-indulgent and decadent life, they kept the world going round. Others did acquire Syphilis, but not to the most dramatic extent. Perhaps it was their mind enabling a modest and disciplined lifestyle which saved them. Perhaps it was sexual prudence which kept the influences of the miasm to a medial level. And let us not ignore that Syphilis, just as the other miasms, nevertheless had some positive effects which helped the human species to carry on.

---

76 Workowski KA and Berman SM. CDC sexually transmitted diseases treatment guidelines. Clin Infect Dis. 2002 Oct 15; 35:S135-7

77 Centers for Disease Control and Prevention. Primary and secondary syphilis among men who have sex with men--New York City, 2001; MMWR Morb Mortal Wkly Rep. 27; 51(38):853-

The Benefits of Syphilis

We already discussed that Syphilis tamed the Sycotic beast. As such it was most beneficial as Sycosis had the tendency to leave all reason and restraint behind. There was one Roman Emperor who actually had unwitting spectators thrown into the arena and eaten by ferocious beasts. Christians being devoured by tigers had become so yesterday... In short, a bit of Syphilis as we defined it above was not a bad thing.

(If at this point you say "but he was obviously Syphilitic, not Sycotic" reconsider: Syphilis was concerned with acts of purification – cruelty was seen as necessity, however regrettable; a sort of collateral occurrence. Sycosis, on the other hand, uses cruelty as stimulation or entertainment. The Emperor was bored, and therefore Sycotic.)

But back to the benefits of Syphilis, the Miasm.

It may be hard to see, but the benefits of this horrendous miasm are in its ability to employ the mind for the purpose of finding truth, faith, divine beauty, knowledge and wisdom. The Syphilitic's mind at its best is highly analytic, deeply concentrated and servile in its devotion to whatever subject it chooses. It drives itself on in endless pursuit, be it theological, philosophical, literary, musical or scientific to come up with the most ingenious works of academic and artistic nature that humankind has ever and probably ever will achieve. Dante's Divine Comedy, Kant's Critique of Pure Reason, Michelangelo's Judgement Day and Wagner's Ring Cycle are all such examples, as are scientific groundbreakers such as Copernicanism and Newton's Theory of Gravitation. It is precisely these examples of Syphilis in all its glory which in the end freed the human species from its (Syphilitic) chains. This is because the unexpected and surprising end result of all noble Syphilitic pursuit was the application of reason over dogma.

In the early 1700s the chains of religious dogma and all it had represented were loosened and gradually replaced by...

Globalisation

The Scientific Revolution

With the understanding that the earth was not the centre of the universe, but an insignificant speck of dust within it, came the inevitable split of science from religion. Strangely, or rather very logically according to what we have written above, most of the newly emerging scientists remained devout to their faith. Science itself, though, took off in the opposite direction and left behind all that was not empirical, mathematical and measurable or firmly rooted in evidence and logic. The Syphilitic mind, split off from the Syphilitic body it inhabited, now created another separate compartment into which all that was ethereal, immaterial and unscientific was placed.

For the common folk no explanation was possible as how one could believe in creation and at the same time accept that Darwin was correct. They carried on wondering and many lost their faith, not being able to reconcile the two. For academics and scholars, everything was still quite in order, as their mind now understood all religious matters to be metaphors, the basic messages of which still applied in the modern world. This allowed them to carry on with their scientific quest.

The quest was not directed towards a specific goal, but took off in all directions. Looking back it seems that, liberated from the ties of religious dogma, humanity now burst forth fuelled by pent-up energy, boundless curiosity and thirst for exploration of the material contents of our world. The search went further and further into detail, but also encompassed the larger phenomena of our world such as the solar system and beyond. Within three centuries humans learnt to harvest on a large scale the energy of steam, coal, gas, oil and the split atom, more recently adding water, wind and solar energies to their repertory of energy sources.

What happened to our miasms meanwhile? As we said, Syphilis enabled this progress to take off by allowing academic knowledge to become advanced enough to end religious dogmatism. Interestingly, we see again an aspect of self-destruction in the way Syphilitic progress led to its own downfall. However, once released from dogma, a new attitude emerged, governed by reason and leaving behind collateral cruelty and the need for discipline. The reasonable mind could begin embracing the previously suppressed physical urges and explain them scientifically. Since on the one hand there was no more God to chastise us for those Sycotic urges and on the other hand we had a scientific explanation for them (or at least we believed there must be one), we began relaxing a little and accepting ourselves more, warts and all.

Thinkers like Siegmund Freud opened the door to the possibility that we were not evil by birth, but that our earliest experiences may have shaped us and our behaviour. In the extreme, past-life therapists believe that previous incarnations of our souls may have experienced trauma that still shapes us today. And homeopaths believe that miasms are part of the story that shapes a person and his actions.

Whilst none of these examples can be seen as scientific or empirical examples of the new world view that has emerged since Syphilis, nevertheless they are part of the way humans experience the world today. Although the transition from Syphilis to our present attitude was mostly driven by science and scientific thinking, the new world view – as we will see below – is not entirely empirical.

In time, specialisation into separate scientific disciplines became more pronounced, new disciplines emerged, and interestingly, the application of the discoveries moved society on towards greater unity. Trains, ships, aeroplanes and cars reduced journey times, bringing the continents as close as half a days' worth of travel. In peak Syphilitic times in Europe, half a day's journey on horseback might have taken a medieval knight only 20 miles down the road. Nowadays we can cross the Atlantic by lunchtime.

And so the scientific quest led us through the French revolution via the industrial revolution to two world wars and beyond, into the age of the computer.

Globalisation and the Age of Reason

At the beginning of the new millennium we see a truly global community within our reach. The official (!) dominant western and eastern world view is one of equality amongst the nations, races and genders.

Yes, we see terrible and most perverted incarnations of Syphilis in African civil wars and in central and South American drug wars. We also witness it in fundamentalist Islamic terror acts. These are societies or parts of societies which have not yet made the transformation from Syphilis to the new age.

The rest of the world is in the grip of globalisation. The advent of the internet and the IT revolution have swiftly transported us into a life where physical distance and differences between people are often irrelevant. Deeply tarnished by Syphilis and its dogmatism, we have liberated ourselves and now live by the law of benign tolerance. We have seen that eradicating differences by force leads nowhere and cannot be sustained. Now we judiciously apply tolerance as an ideal, and this works much better – as long as we each do an equal amount of tolerating.

We employ our reason to decide what is best.

In a way, we have lost our edges and extremes. The corners have been knocked out of us. We do not struggle through life; our aim is to float along. We avoid sharp lefts and rights and look for a gently curving middle path.

We eliminated the seesaw of indulgence and purgatory simply by breaking through dogma with reason.

The Nature of Reason

Let us look at this process more closely. Whilst Syphilis occupied itself with fencing off 'lower' parts of the inner human existence and employing dogma and harsh discipline to tame the Sycotic beast, the new age tries to dissolve conflict with reason. This means that we are still up in our minds, but to a great extent we are using logic and scientific knowledge to solve problems. Instead of blindly following rules in order to avoid punishment, we ask questions and answer them by looking at all sides of the argument. Reason requires non-bias and lack of personal investment in the outcome. A decision is arrived at because the facts indicate that it will be the best path for everyone involved.

The transition from Syphilis to the next miasm was only possible because some very advanced Syphilitic thinkers discovered facts about the world that shattered the status quo. These people were unique in their make-up or lucky in their personal circumstances in that they did not fear punishment for tearing down dogma.

To begin with, we need to thank Copernicus. Around 1540, his revolutionary theory of heliocentrism was actually received with delight by the then ruling Pope, but some 70 years later was proclaimed heresy by another one.

Heresy or not, the idea that the sun did not move around the Earth took the wind out of the Syphilitic sail and opened the door for reason to take over.

Slowly, other scientific explorations took place and a new breed of scholars emerged who did not just discuss whether the wine taken at holy communion was the actual blood of Christ or indeed only a representation of it, but who asked questions about the physiology of the human body, about chemical and biochemical processes, pathology, infectious diseases and generally about physical and mathematical problems. Of course this type of academic pursuit had always existed, but now, as dogma crumbled, the door had been opened for the inquisitive and liberated mind to take charge in a major way.

Strangely enough, many such scholars occupied themselves with physical life, i.e. the human body. This body, which had been viewed as a source of urges to be repressed for so long, now re-emerged as a valid subject of discussion. We remained children of Syphilis in that we talked about the body only from a purely functional point of view. But still, this discussion and exploration led, and still leads, to many findings that allow us to understand ourselves and what we need to lead a healthy life. In this way, the human body was reinstated as important and something we pay attention to.

By the end of the 20th century, the scientific quest had become universal. What was undertaken by a handful of scholars in isolation 300 years ago, now was being pursued by a countless number of people at thousands of universities and research centres around the globe.

At this point in our discussion we must understand the importance of science and factual thinking in human social evolution. It was only – and I repeat only – the scientific quest and the thirst for knowledge about how the world works from a mechanical angle that has enabled us to liberate ourselves from the Syphilitic age. Without scientific discoveries, the house of cards that enabled the European monotheistic societies to function would not have come tumbling down. It was necessary to de-mystify life in order to liberate ourselves from fear of the unknown. We did not only fear God, we also still did not know why we got ill, why the weather was unkind, what brought about the seasons, why we got pregnant, etc. All these unexplained but everyday phenomena kept us in a space of insecurity and worry. And as we remember from the beginning of our discussion, man wanted to escape his constant anxieties.

Looking back, the survival anxieties of pre-Psoric man had not really been solved at all. We still feared the weather, the seasons, the plague, God and other human beings. All that had changed was the environment we lived in. It was more comfortable (for a decisive number of people) and it had allowed an enormous expansion of population size.

To make another attempt at conquering our primal anxiety, it was important to put religion and all its inexplicable details into a separate box and move the rest of our understanding on. Every single scientific fact that has been established so far, and will be established, furthermore helps us in this quest. Instead of blindly following rules because we fear punishment, we ask questions and answer them by looking at all sides of the argument. This means we employ our reason. As I said above, the term reason implies non-bias and lack of personal investment in the outcome. A decision is arrived at because the facts indicate that it will be the best alternative for everyone involved.

In turn, reason allows us to remain factual and scientific (although this is not necessarily helpful in the long run – more about this later).

However much we adore science and however much we believe in our non-biased mind calmly dissecting facts and arriving at "reasonable" decisions, the reality for most individuals looks quite different. As we discussed before, apart from our thinking mind, nature has bestowed us with a feeling body. Since the advent of reason and all the factual discoveries, we are not as appalled by our body and its feelings anymore; in fact we find ourselves rather interested. When enlightenment began, not only mechanical facts were gathered, but also philosophical discussions about the meaning of life and the purpose of human existence became quite fashionable. These discussions necessarily led to a branching out into the more subjective areas of our existence, i.e. how an individual felt, responded, and coped with certain scenarios and circumstances.

By the beginning of the 20th century Siegmund Freud was ready to father a new branch of academic pursuit – psychoanalysis. Thanks to Freud, the occupation with emotions and their influence on our subjective and very personal experience of life became extremely fashionable. So much so that nowadays most people would agree that some amount of emotional awareness and self-development would be beneficial, perhaps even essential, for leading a happy and productive/constructive life.

This insight is rather important, because it means that factual and scientific decision-making is not the only way by which human beings operate. They also use their emotions.

The idea of Emotional Intelligence is one of the newer models that try to describe this process. Humans differ in their ability to perceive, use, understand and manage emotions. The more proficient a person is in each area, the more successful their social interactions will be. Since everything in life depends on successful social interactions on some level, even at the workplace, emotional intelligence becomes one of the most important aspects of our being. As homeopaths we would support this idea in its totality. A person aware of their inhibitions is more able to work at letting them go than someone who is unaware and does not know where to begin seeking help. Many unhealthy compensation behaviours such as smoking and drinking are fuelled by emotional instabilities, and a higher degree of emotional intelligence allows a person to process his underlying emotional imbalance and reduce the compensatory behaviour. Ultimately, the decision to stop smoking must be taken by the factual mind (which, informed by science, knows that smoking is dangerous) and the emotionally intelligent mind (which has realised that the habit is maintained by insecurity) letting go of unhelpful feelings.

It is definitely a hallmark of the new age to acknowledge and attempt an integration of emotions and the reasoning mind into our governing operating mechanisms. Thus the new age has not only brought us facts in order to be reasonable, but also allowed emotions to be considered as informants of reason.

Unfortunately, many people are not proficient in processing their emotions in a helpful way and this can for some become a major problem. Although theoretically most people would subscribe to the idea of emotional intelligence and its importance, in practice they are unable to apply the process. A more Sycotic person might secretly wish they could manage their emotions maturely, but publicly ridicule anyone trying to do so in the hope of being amusing and therefore popular. A more Syphilitic person would ignore the existence of their emotions or drown them by force (alcohol, drugs, punishment). A person firmly rooted in 'The New Age' will believe they are processing their emotions maturely, but all that is taking place is a glossing over. This is because in this New Age all must be nice, kind and easy, coated with sugar and love. Negative emotions are briefly allowed but then all that is ugly and imperfect will be smoothed over.

The reason for this is partly to do with the following.

Tolerance

The spirit of the new age is one of tolerance, freedom, kindness and charity. At least this is how the more economically secure nations would define their overall mentality.

Again it is empirical knowledge which has brought us to this, as through advances in travel, energy production and IT technologies, physical distance has become irrelevant to a great degree. As interactions became faster, they also became more efficient. Information media became fashionable and radios, tvs, and now computers served to bring people closer together. Never before could we see in moving pictures how a person was shot in an action of civil war or how another starved in a refugee camp. Since humans respond more to visual stimulation than the written word, individuals separated by oceans became aware of each others' plight. Being shown pictures of human suffering on a regular basis, a critical mass of individuals around the globe became less self-absorbed and more charitable, first only in theory, but more and more also in their actions.

What happened simultaneously was an ethical shift away from nationalistic thinking, racism and gender discrimination (at least in theory) towards a mingling of the sexes, skin colours and creeds at the workplace and in private life. Of course there is a long way to go yet to a complete disappearance of discrimination, but at least in our minds and feelings we strive towards this ideal.

Paradoxically, the two world wars were the driving force behind this development towards a kinder and more charitable world. The US and associated satellite economies were propelled to superpower status and thus became able to fund the exponential explosion of empirical knowledge. In addition and of equal importance was the unanimous abhorrence of the holocaust as well as the terrible events during and following the Russian Revolution. These brought about an adoption of the only possible post-holocaust and post-Stalin stance: non-racism, non-discrimination, freedom of speech and gender equality. It was as if the horrific extremes seen in the first half of the 20th century brought about a general sobering, stock-taking and full embrace of a truly humane attitude. The term 'ethics' comes to mind and the ethical stance taken from the mid-20th century onwards by many individuals and society as a whole very much describes our present mentality.

The above applies to the non-communist and economically developed societies only. Behind the iron curtain and in large parts of Africa, Asia and South America a more Syphilitic stance prevailed. But it is the economically more developed societies which drive social evolution forward and so we will discuss the new attitude they adapted as an example of the next miasm.

Thus scientific progress as well as the apocalyptic Syphilitic events of the 20th century brought about the new age of tolerance, kindness, freedom of speech and gender equality.

All is One

In line with globalisation on a technical as well as emotional level, we also see in this new age a resurgence of the spiritual.

For many more traditionally aligned people this means returning to their Christian faith, even if we see a more varied approach with many different evangelical and protestant sects gaining popularity. Whereas during Syphilitic times religion was a means of imposing discipline, in this new age it is an expression of the new spirit of tolerance which teaches that all are equal, and that remaining controversy can be overcome by tolerance and kindness. The idea that God is charitable and benevolent prevails and nobody is talking about or afraid of eternal damnation or purgatory at this point. Nowadays we go to church to express our need for community and perhaps to find our sense of community.

The new Bahai faith expresses exactly this and it is expanding to become a major religion in the new millennium. Interestingly, the Bahai faith is strongly rooted in Islam, but also takes in many aspects of Christianity and Judaism. In this way it is a truly "New Age religion", bridging all differences and finding unity in the essential message of charity and community values.

For the more adventurous citizen of a non-communist and economically advanced society, Buddha and the various sects of Hinduism have much to offer. The idea of karma, rebirth and charity in Hinduism, but more so the theory of eternal bliss issued from Buddha seem attractive to an ethically minded and harmony-seeking individual. Hinduism itself is peaceful, liberal and extremely tolerant, with the idea of heresy being completely absent. Whilst Hinduism is considered the oldest religion on Earth, it is equally a religion for the new age.

Buddha, who has taken Hinduism a step further, represents our new miasm perfectly. Eternal bliss is not found in happiness, as feeling happy means you will need to feel sad later; this is the law of balance or duality. Bliss (not to be confused with happiness), can on the other hand be found only by letting go of all needs. When you let go, you get off the proverbial see-saw all humans find themselves sitting on. Buddha realised that being human means being suspended in duality, a state where good is always balanced by bad, night by day, laughter by tears. Buddha found that it is possible to transcend this state of duality and let go of it.

The Zen proverb "Before enlightenment: chopping wood, carrying water; after enlightenment: chopping wood, carrying water" expresses what happens to us once we have found bliss. Life just carries on as before, but we do not suffer any ups and downs anymore. We just are. We do not put any value on anything and we live in the present only. Anxiety, remember, only comes when we look forward or dwell on the past. Since all we wanted to escape from at the beginning of our journey, and ever since, was anxiety, it seems therefore that with the advent of the new age we have finally reached our destination – a possibility of redemption, a possibility of cure.

Unfortunately, for most of us in this century, Buddhism remains a vague idea.

It is again science which has sparked another development, a type of spiritual conviction without name or congregation, but nevertheless not too far removed in ideology from any of the others. This proclaims a connection of all individuals or even all living organisms on a particle level. Phenomena such as telepathy as well as synchronicity between people separated in locality have fuelled this. This connection is not just on a consciousness level but also found on the level of basic material. Equally, it is not only contemporary, but also bridges time and space.

The idea that atoms cannot naturally be destroyed, just recycled into different compounds, leads on to the realisation that our own body may contain atoms that were once part of a tyrannosaurus rex or a primeval bacteria. Having negative attitudes towards other living organisms or even other elements in our world would therefore ultimately harm ourselves. The movie "Avatar" was a perfect expression of this, where humans and other organisms could connect at will and exchange information for the common good.

For some, this type of spirituality seems shallow and pseudo-scientific, but for others it still makes sense on a very basic level. It teaches us to be careful in our actions and judgements, as all is one.

A New Miasm

Whilst the new age with its ethical convictions is definitely an improvement from Syphilitic dogma and has brought a sense of liberation and peace to large parts of the world, we simultaneously are witness to ever deepening disease states and even to new, more virulent infections.

Thus, the story of miasm as a saviour of the human species but killer of the individual continues.

In order to survive Syphilis we had to once more rethink and regroup. The outcome is an ethically-minded society that is set for an exponential scientific and technological roller-coaster of development. The price we pay as individuals is to fall victim to the deepest states of disease where a life without pharmaceutical support becomes impossible.

So what has gone wrong now?

Cancer, the Ultimate Multi-factorial Problem

At this point in time, the newly found spirit of tolerance and universal kindness remains very much an ideal and a theoretical value which we strive for and believe our lives should be governed by. But in fact it is as if we are covering our existence with a universal sugar coating to make it more palatable.

Underneath this agreeable vision of sweetness, peace and love, Syphilis and all the other miasms are still raging their war, so much so that in almost every action of any human being at any time we see aspects, attitudes and motives belonging to any previous miasm playing their part and lending the new miasm their particular flavour.

Wherever we look, we see corruption, greed, one-upmanship, crime, slander, cynicism, addiction and depression to name a few examples of negative human behaviour.

I believe that the discrepancy between what we strive for and what we do comes about because of too many factors affecting us at any one time. So much so that we are not free to make reasonable (i.e. "good for everyone involved") decisions, even if we wanted to.

A good, but relatively mild, example would be the ethically minded investor – such as any homeopath should be. Imagine the unlikely possibility of having £100,000 to spare and wanting to invest it in stocks and shares. We may do the necessary research ourself or use a broker, but in any case we will end up comparing ethical funds with non-ethical funds. The sad truth is that ethical funds do not perform as well, because they do not invest in arms, food or pharmaceuticals, these three being the most unethical but best-performing funds available. What do we do? Throw our money out of the window and invest ethically? Or do we turn a blind eye and become an accomplice in our government's war on innocent civilians, or the GM and pharmaceutical industry's attempts to produce sick, drug-dependent people?

In our aim to be ethical, to be kind, to be charitable, to consider everyone involved, can we truly be sure we are doing the right thing?

Another example would be the ethical shopper. Is it even possible to be ethically correct when purchasing anything from food to household goods to cars and books? Of course not. Too many factors are involved. Too many pieces in the chain of production. Too many people to consider. And still, at the end of the day, we need to be able to afford the product we need to buy.

My point is that our lives have become complicated. Too many factors interplay and blur the picture. There is no black and white anymore, just shades of grey. Sometimes it is hard to find our way through, however much we try to retain our decency and integrity.

Interestingly, as homeopaths we recognise a parallel in one of the symptom pictures we would use the Cancer nosode for and, as it happens, we see many people in this state. This is when the patient presents with a large variety of symptoms that belong to different totalities. It is in such a patient as if too many factors have affected him in his lifetime and they have all blurred the picture into an out-of-focus mess. The Cancer nosode may be used to benefit in such a case.

Another aspect of the multi-factorial character of this miasm is seen in the way it is so transparent and without character of its own. It takes on, or rather lets shine through so easily, all previous miasmatic influences, be they in attitude, behaviour or in biochemical problems.

In our practice we often see Cancer with a Syphilitic slant (perhaps producing anorexia), or Cancer with a Tubercular taste (perhaps a respiratory pathology), or a Sycotic Cancer (very poorly disciplined). Even Psora can flavour Cancer, as we see in many hay fever cases.

The blandness of this miasm is found in some ways also in the attitude we discussed. When we aim to be kind, to be tolerant of and charitable to everyone, we necessarily must give up some of the more dominant or clearly defining characteristics of ourselves. This is because it works both ways. We also wish others to be kind to us and we can expect to be treated this way only if we are somewhat lacking edges and corners.

Emotional Suppression

Homeopaths believe it is possible to suppress emotions, and we mostly mean negative emotions. This idea is similar to the model of the subconscious in psychotherapy/analysis, which is supposed to contain any negative emotions we have not processed. The problem is that these emotions still influence our behaviour and attitudes and can cause disease, emotional, mental or physical.

When we look at our miasmatic history, emotional suppression in line with this above model only really started in a major way during Syphilitic times. The body as the seat of feelings was denied any importance and was generally neglected in any person affected by the Syphilitic miasm. This was one reason for the deepening of chronic disease.

The new age reinstated the body and its feelings to centre stage. We are allowed to feel and discuss our emotions, but we are also required to be kind, compassionate and polite at all times. As discussed above this necessarily leads to a giving up of anything that might upset another or be too controversial.

Another aspect of new age reason is that only a mature person can be expected to be reasonable. The art of non-biased argumentation and non-investment in the outcome of any discussion is something only a few people attain. But we are all expected to be masters in this and, what's more, we are expecting our children to know it too.

Average middle-class children of age 5 or over are expected to resolve conflict non-violently, explain their feelings and understand action and consequence. It is of course good to aim for this, but all too often parents train their children to attain these qualities too soon in life, when a natural exuberance and spontaneity should prevail. It is questionable whether a child can tell the difference between loud angry screaming, or loud happy screaming. Children will just assume that screaming per se is not allowed and with this, the expression of happiness is forbidden too. Thus children learn at a young age that the open expression of feelings, positive or negative, is frowned upon. They learn to hide their feelings. And in the spirit of Cancer, they believe they must hide their feelings so as not to offend or upset others.

Looking at how emotions are handled we can identify three pathways that are commonly used.

One is to become aware of an emotion and successfully eliminate it. In the case of children this looks like laughing, crying, screaming, sulking, hitting etc. In this way the emotion is eliminated, just as vomiting eliminates some disagreeable food item. So letting a child cry until they have finished would be an example of this. The process of elimination stops by itself when it has finished. In this way the emotion does not have any impact on us and does not become suppressed or hidden. No compensatory behaviour is necessary.

Adults have to a great extent lost this ability to eliminate their emotions because some ways of venting emotions are socially unacceptable (hitting, screaming) and often adults have gone through the process of learning to hide their emotions and so are not able to vent them. In some situations and environments even adults can go through this child-like elimination process safely and in an accepted way. But even if this is not possible in all instances, there are other ways to eliminate emotions healthily and these include talking about them in a safe environment.

A second and perhaps almost as ideal a way of processing and eliminating feelings would be to stay quiet and observe the actual feeling in one's body. Interestingly, when we just watch the feeling, we will find that it passes. It will take a little while, but it will pass. At that point we have successfully eliminated the emotion.

A third way, most commonly used, is the hiding of the emotion and this is seen more with older children (age 7 or so upwards) and adults. The person remains aware of how they are feeling but cannot vent it in any way for whatever reason. In many instances of this happening, unless a person is aware that feelings pass by themselves and knows how to take advantage of this mechanism, a compensatory behaviour becomes necessary that acts to numb or drown the uncomfortable feeling saturating our body. Eating sugary treats, drinking alcohol and using drugs to numb those feelings we cannot vent, serve their purpose, but make us ill in other ways if indulged in too often. And this, in my opinion, is the most common route by which emotional suppression becomes a cause of disease. The need to suppress the emotion is the susceptibility (the attitude to be socially acceptable) and the use of substances to numb the feeling makes us physically ill.

Some people will say that the very act of numbing an emotion causes disease because the feeling has not been eliminated and is still somewhere in our memory, subconscious or other place in our body/mind/spirit. This may be so, but we have no evidence of this, so I prefer to give a more plausible explanation. Using health-eroding substances to manage emotions is obviously damaging to our bodies and in itself enough to make us ill.

There may be a fourth (not scientifically verifiable) way we process emotions and this is when we commit extremely traumatic memories and feelings to our subconscious and away from our active memory. This is to protect ourselves and make it possible to lead a relatively normal life. Victims of extreme abuse are said to use this type of emotional management. In this case, the emotion is probably still having an enormous effect on the life and health of the individual. But just as the physical body can encapsulate a diseased area and therefore stop it from having an effect on the rest of the body, I believe the mind can do this too. And so perhaps a truly successful suppression of extreme negative emotions is not a disadvantage, but a benefit – at least in the short term.

However, on the whole it is my view that most emotions, whether hidden or not, only produce disease if a compensatory behaviour acts as a stimulus. Only the marriage of susceptibility and stimulus produces disease.

Harmony, or the Susceptibility to Cancer

As discussed above, one of the susceptibilities for the Cancer miasm is the need to be kind and tolerant and the matching stimulus for this susceptibility is the drowning of negative emotions and urges in toxic substances that in the long run produce physical disease. Interestingly, the substances used (sugar, alcohol, tobacco, drugs) produce predominantly diabetes and cancer (two diseases which dominate the cancer miasm from a homeopath's point of view). These substances have to be used over a long time in order to be harmful, but since every human on this planet has inherited all previous miasms, our health is not in the best state to start with, even before we begin to poison ourselves.

Just as with the other miasms, Cancer, the miasm, has many stimuli. Some are emotional, some are mental and some are lifestyle related and so of physical or rather chemical nature.

What is new in this miasm is that it also has multiple susceptibilities, although loosely related.

One such susceptibility is the need to be perfect. Actually, this arises from the need to be kind and tolerant at all times (a type of emotional perfection), but extends to physical and academic perfection. The new age demands of people to be on top of developments and to keep abreast of all innovation. The speed of expansion of knowledge is such that only the most capable, bright and ambitious persons will stand out. Anyone remotely average will be left behind.

This forces parents to push their children relentlessly into earlier and earlier academic achievements, so much so that recently in the UK a curriculum for toddlers was issued. And we do not need to get good grades only in academic subjects. No, we need also to be good at tennis, dancing, piano playing, drama, judo, etc. In other words, an all-round genius is just about good enough.

Perfectionism is a very pronounced trait of the Cancer miasm. It is met with a mixture of stimuli. One is workoholism, which produces adrenal burn out similar to that caused by fear (see Syphilis). Another is stress relief through toxic substances such as sugar, alcohol, drugs etc. We see a lot of this behaviour in middle-class adolescents.

Another very important stimulus meeting the susceptibility of perfectionism is control of food intake in order to become physically perfect. Anorexia is partially Syphilitic (self-destructive) but also part of the cancer picture because the individual desires to be beautiful and visually perfect. In addition, many do not seem to suffer when they do not eat, but somehow manage to suppress any physically uncomfortable feelings and even get a kick out of starving themselves.

The attitude of perfectionism is also met with fastidiousness as a stimulus. This reaches from cleanliness and order to punctuality, germ phobia and obsessive compulsive disorders. The spectrum of fastidiousness has strong roots in Sycosis, because the Sycotic person desires to control himself (but cannot do it) and is disgusted by his dirt and mess. As a next step, fastidiousness is encouraged by Syphilis, as a backlash against the Sycotic chaos. Especially in this miasm any bodily secretions are thought of as disgusting and any trace of them must be completely removed. In the new age, this attitude has led to a spectrum of wide-spread fastidiousness as described above. Of course, when it is mild, it is just a little difficult to live with. But germ-phobia can lead to disease if we compensate by using too many chemical cleaners, detergents and soaps. These are highly toxic and can in the long run cause disease. In fact most of the chemicals used in detergents and soaps are carcinogenic. We will discuss this in more depth later.

The other way germ-phobia leads to disease is if we become overly worried about acute or chronic illness, and this is where perfectionism as an attitude/susceptibility meets another set of stimuli. If we believe that germs can kill regardless of the immune system's ability to fight them, we have lost the battle against chronic disease. This is because we then will feel the need to use antibiotics and other pharmaceuticals as soon as something is not quite right. Our immune system will never exert itself, and therefore become weaker. In turn our bodies become so fragile that we really do need pharmaceuticals for every little problem. And most pharmaceuticals have side-effects which in turn may need more medication. In the end we see a blurred picture of symptoms presenting in a weak body; the hallmark of the Cancer miasm.

Homeopaths believe that the treatment of acute disease with pharmaceuticals increases the risk of developing chronic disease. Since we are all born with the tendency to have chronic ailments (even a conventional scientist would agree with the fact that we all possess genes that predispose to various chronic states), the use of pharmaceuticals is a risk factor and a possible stimulus or trigger. We do not even need to mention the word suppression when we talk about this phenomenon. Pharmaceuticals are man-made chemicals and have side-effects which may or may not include triggering genes that set chronic disease in motion. They also may or may not structurally or functionally damage other body parts (that they were not intended for).[78] Tamoxifen (a breast cancer drug) and several types of chemotherapy are scientifically proven carcinogens.[79] We do not know enough about this subject yet, but my guess is that research in this area is not paid for by pharmaceutical companies (who are the main sponsors of medical research).

So, the susceptibility of perfectionism meets the stimulus of germ-phobia which produces various limitations to our life as well as outright physical and mental disease. Obsessive compulsive disorder is of course the main mental problem arising, and whilst people suffering from this disorder are not physically ill in the first instance they tend to become so as they are limiting their lives more and more. Eventually they do not leave the house, get no fresh air or sunshine, do not exercise, eat only a very limited diet and, as we know, these are all factors leading to chronic ailments as discussed in previous chapters.

It is interesting that from a nutritionist's point of view, a person with obsessive compulsive disorder would be considered either lacking or be highly loaded with certain minerals such as zinc and copper (and this can be due to inherited problems), but equally most probably would be suffering from metal toxicity. As we know, this can also

---

78 Sanborn M, Cole D, et al. Systematic Review of pesticide human health effects. Ontario College of family Physicians. 2004; 1-186.

79 http://monographs.iarc.fr/ENG/Classification/ClassificationsAlphaOrder.pdf; 17th Jan 2012

be inherited[80] and so there is a strong case for pronouncing this disorder miasmatic. Also one would be looking at food allergies and intolerance to chemicals in foods such as preservatives and colourings and a blood sugar balance/insulin metabolism problem. As we have seen, the Psoric person had a tendency to react to grasses. Tuberculinum had widespread inflammation due to arachidonic acid in dairy leading to respiratory and skin symptoms; again a possible allergy. Sycosis added mould and yeast as an allergic trigger. In Cancer we see a tendency to have multiple allergies and reasons for this include the critical mass of man-made chemicals bombarding our systems from conception onwards. We will discuss this more in detail later.

The basic susceptibility of Cancer from which all others derive is the deep yearning for peace and harmony. This desire has been with us ever since we left paradise and acquired self-consciousness. However, after the long-winded chaos of Sycosis and the horrors of Syphilis in the middle ages culminating in the apocalyptic world wars, a critical mass of people were desperate and ready to make their absolute priority lasting peace and harmony amongst the races, nations, genders and creeds.

The primal anxiety around food supply and safety from animals and the elements had, during Sycosis and Syphilis, expanded to fear of cruelty from other human beings. In this new age, all we desire is to get rid of all anxiety and fear and so in true homeopathic manner we remove the latest fear first and make peace amongst fellow human beings our priority.

---

80 Crinnion WJ. Maternal levels of xenobiotics that affect fetal development and childhood health. Altern Med Rev. 2009 Sep; 14(3):212-22.

As a second step we secure the food supply by making it as independent from weather, soil condition and pests as possible. Of course, our newly found scientific expertise alone makes this possible. We invent fertilizers, pesticides and preservatives. We also enjoy superb storage and transport so that absolutely nobody in the economically developed nations (and this is where the Cancer miasm is active) needs to go hungry. Of course deep down we still have financial worries, but this is a different issue. As such, the food supply is as secure as it can be on this planet. (Lately we have seen droughts and floods as well as soil erosion and depletion. We also worry about population size in relation to food supply. These problems revive our primal anxieties.)

A further step is the victory over acute disease. This deserves its own chapter, but for now we will just say that we have more or less eradicated death from acute disease (in first world countries) and we also have conquered many states of pain and suffering due to chronic disease. This does not mean we truly cure, but it means we know how to relieve pain, remove germs, regulate out-of-order metabolisms and extend lives with the help of pharmaceuticals and medical procedures. Again, we can only thank science for this.

The list goes on, but for now we have said enough to show what effect the desire for harmony and peace has had in our times.

The problem with this attitude/susceptibility is that:
    a)   it leads to behaviours that act as disease stimuli,
    b)   it is very difficult to attain in our present situation.

159

For example: pesticides, fertilizers and preservatives lead to soil depletion and poisoning of the environment as well as of those who eat foods treated with it. This cannot be called harmony (because we created other problems by using these chemicals) and so we have not reached our goal. Often we solve one problem, but inadvertently create another one, as in the case of the pesticide example. Apart from being toxic to us, pesticides interrupt the food chain and so we will suffer in the long run.

Another example would be the use of antibiotics to overcome pain and suffering in our children's ear infections. We solve one problem, but are likely to create disharmony in the digestive system, liver and immune system. The need to eradicate suffering causes a behaviour that creates more suffering.

Of course it is thanks to science that we can save lives, but it is also thanks to science that we are in a position to abuse it. There are better alternatives available (just as in the case with solving primal anxiety and Buddhism) but not enough people know about them. A critical mass has not yet been reached.

As with all previous miasms, the Cancer miasm has a clear susceptibility/attitude and matching disease stimuli that go with it. This time around, disease ensues because the attitude can never be truly practised and brought to fruition. It is impossible to always be in harmony; it is impossible to always be kind; it is impossible to be perfect. What we see, instead of a realisation of the attitude, is compensatory behaviour that helps us cover up or get through as easily as possible when we have failed to satisfy our original aim. And this compensation leads to disease.

We see this mechanism at work in the emotional sphere when, instead of having it out with our best friend, we reach for the bottle and feel much better after 2-3 glasses, but our liver, bowels and brain suffer. We see it in the mental sphere when instead of resting we push ourselves to study, work and perform in order to be successful and "perfect", but our adrenal glands, blood sugar balance and fertility suffer. And we see it in the physical sphere, when we use painkillers to stop the headache instead of drinking more water or cutting out dairy, but our gut lining suffers.

On a grand scale we have become reliant on comfort and speed to achieve ease of living – again a type of harmony and beauty. Chemical cleaners, weed killers, kitchen appliances, cordless phones, wireless computers, cars, painkillers, antibiotics etc etc. Wherever you turn, our life has been arranged so that we do not struggle physically, and expend as little energy and time as possible on menial tasks and sick leave. The struggle is over – we float through life on a cloud of pink candy. Dirt dissolves within seconds, weeds disintegrate in front of our eyes, rubbish is taken out of our sight, infections resolve in 24 hours. Life is wonderful and easy.

But Cancer is sneaky. Underneath all the harmony, ease and beauty it works away unnoticed. Those chemicals which dissolve the dirt in your bathtub cause lung cancer in those who breathe them in too often. Those chemicals that kill your dandelions cause cancer in those who breathe them in or touch them too often. They also leach into the water supply and in spite of the municipal water work's efforts end up to some degree in your drinking water causing cancer. Those chemicals that leach from your rubbish into the soil and subsequently into the water table, also end up in your body by the same route. They also end up in your lungs, because some rubbish is incinerated.

Luckily our bodies seem to have a threshold or tolerance level for toxins, but once this has been breached, anything can happen. Perhaps the worst aspect of this is that because of the elapsed time and the lack of odour and invisibility of toxins we do not even realise what is making us ill and so we cannot learn or protect ourselves.

The Ethical Vegetarian

There is another variant to the attitude of tolerance and desire for harmony, and this one is particularly trouble-some, because we have no satisfactory solution of the dilemma we find ourselves in. I am talking about ethical vegetarianism combined with a passionate concern for the environment. The two often go together.

In essence, the ethical vegetarian is giving preference to the life of animals over her own. In order to not be part of inhumane animal husbandry, she chooses to eat plant protein and dairy, eggs, plus an extraordinary amount of cereals. But surely, you say, this is a good thing?

Ethically, as a mature human being, nobody would argue with refusing to eat inhumanely reared animals. Most of us respect and perhaps sometimes wish we could also be as steadfast as our vegetarian friends. We turn our heads in horror when walking past abattoirs and we do not wish to know what happens inside a factory farm. But strangely, most of us still eat meat. We somehow manage to override our reservations and tuck into bacon, steak and fish pie, regardless of where it came from. (To be fair, many meat eaters will chose organic fare and so avoid at least some of the ethically questionable issues.)

We therefore notice that a majority of people have an overwhelming need to eat animal flesh. No measure of campaigning against it will convince them to give it up.

The reason may be that human beings simply have no alternative.

It is mostly the question of obtaining sufficient protein which comes to mind, but there are also other issues such as iron deficiency and lack of Vitamin B12 that are being raised by opponents to vegetarianism.

In line with our story so far, I would single out the protein dilemma to be the most difficult to solve. Vegetarians rely on dairy, eggs, soy and combining cereals and pulses to obtain all essential amino acids from their protein sources. (Proteins are made up of amino acids. Eight of these cannot be assembled from others and so have to be eaten regularly.) Going back to Psora and Tuberculosis, we have already extensively discussed how cereals and dairy and to some extent pulses damage our gut and cause systemic problems that extend to the brain and the even the mind and emotions.[81] This means that three vegetarian sources

81 Kitts DD, Weiler K. Bioactive proteins and peptides from food sources. Applications of bioprocesses used in isolation and recovery. Curr Pharm Des. 2003; 9(16):1309-23

Teschemacher H. Opioid receptor ligands derived from food proteins. Curr Pharm Des. 2003; 9(16):1331-44.

Askenazi et al. Immunologic reaction of psychotic patients to fractions of gluten. AmJ Psychiatry 1979; 136:1306-1309

Hibbeln J. Fish Consumption and major depression. Lancet,vol.351, April 18, 1998. p.1213

Tanskanen Antti et al. Fish consumption, depression and suicidal tendency in a general population. Archives of general psychiatry, Vol. 58, May 2011; pp.512-13

Sioudrou et al. Opioid peptides derived from food proteins. The exorphins. J Biol Chem.1979; 254:2446-2449.

Guzyeyeva GV. Lectin glycosylation as a marker of thin gut inflammation. The Faseb Journal. 2008; 22:898.3

Pusztai A. Dietary lectins are metabolic signals for the gut and modulate immune and hormone functions. Eur J Clin Nutr. 1993 Oct; 47(10):691-9.

of essential amino acids bring with it a high risk of developing serious health issues. In particular, eating wheat, a food
heavily relied on by many vegetarians, has detrimental
effects partially due to its component WGA (wheat germ
agglutinin). Issues associated with WGA go beyond the
digestive system and include cytotoxicity, immunotoxicity,
neurotoxicity, cardiotoxicity, endocrine disruption and proinflammatory effects.[82]

The problem is augmented by the need to eat the
offending foods in very high quantities in order to extract
sufficient amounts of the eight essential amino acids. These
are less abundant in plant sources than in animal flesh.

To solve their protein supply issues, vegans in particular
are compelled to add another source of trouble to their
diet – soy.

Soy contains the complete set of amino acids, including
the eight essential ones. But we know by now that the question of protein is not only one of quantity, but also one
of quality. We have already discussed the issue of lectins
in pulses, and soy contains a high number of these. Apart
from protein, soy also provides substances which actually

82 Dalla Pellegrina C, Perbellini O et al. Effects of wheat germ agglutinin on
human gastrointestinal epithelium: insights from an experimental model
of immune/epithelial cell interaction. Toxicol Appl Pharmacol. 2009 Jun 1;
237(2):146-53. Epub 2009. Mar 28

Guzyeyeva GV. Lectin glycosylation as a marker of thin gut inflammation. The
FASEB Journal. 200. 22:898.3.

Pusztai A, Ewen SWet al. Antinutritive effects of wheat-germ agglutinin and
other N-acetylglucosamine-specific lectins.Br J Nutr. 1993 Jul;70(1):313-21

Tchernychev B, Wilchek M. Natural human antibodies to dietary lectins. FEBS
Lett. 1996 Nov 18;397(2-3):139-42

Liu WK, Sze SC et al.Wheat germ lectin induces G2/M arrest in mouse L929
fibroblasts. J Cell Biochem. 2004 Apr 15; 91(6):1159-73.

Ohmori T, Yatomi Y et al. Wheat germ agglutinin-induced platelet activation
via platelet endothelial cell adhesion molecule-1: involvement of rapid
phospholipase C gamma 2 activation by Src family kinases. Biochemistry.
2001 Oct 30; 40(43):12992-3001

inhibit the digestion of the very protein it is supposed to supply. These are called trypsin inhibitors and they block the action of enzymes needed for protein digestion. They are not completely inactivated during cooking and can produce chronic amino acid deficiencies.

In addition soy contains a chemical (haemagglutinin) that promotes red blood cells to clump together. This substance (as well as the above mentioned trypsin inhibitors) also stunts growth.

The soy bean has the highest amount of phytate of any eatable plant and these are resistant to cooking. Phytates, as we discussed under Psora, bind to minerals and prevent their absorption. In this way, soy foods contribute to endemic nutritional deficiencies in the third world.[83] Further, soy contains goitrogens. These are substances that negatively affect the thyroid gland and may produce hypothyroid conditions.[84]

Aware of the anti-nutritional properties of soy, the soy industry has come up with soy protein isolate (SPI) to remove the substances in question. This product is the main ingredient in many vegetarian protein substitutes

---

83 Van Rensburg et al., Nutritional status of African populations predisposed to esophageal cancer, Nutrition and Cancer, vol. 4, 1983, pp. 206-216;

Moser, P.B. et al., Copper, iron, zinc and selenium dietary intake and status of Nepalese lactating women and their breastfed infants, American Journal of Clinical Nutrition 47:729-734, April 1988;

Harland, B.F. et al. Nutritional status and phytate: zinc and phytate X calcium: zinc dietary molar ratios of lacto-ovovegetarian Trappist monks: 10 years later, Journal of the American Dietetic Association 88:1562-1566, December 1988.

84 Ishizuki, Y. et al. The effects on the thyroid gland of soybeans administered experimentally in healthy subjects, Nippon Naibunpi Gakkai Zasshi. 1991; 767:622-629.

Divi, R.L. et al. Anti-thyroid isoflavones from the soybean. Biochemical Pharmacology. 1997; 54:1087-1096.

Cassidy, A. et al. Biological Effects of a Diet of Soy Protein Rich in Isoflavones on the Menstrual Cycle of Premenopausal Women. American Journal of Clinical Nutrition; 1994, 60:333-340.

such as veggie sausages, burgers, fake cheeses, and even baby formula.

Unfortunately they have thrown out the baby with the bath water, as much of the desirable protein, especially the amino acid lysine, is denatured during the process. This means that most of the protein becomes inaccessible by our system.[85]

In addition, many fake-meat products are flavoured with MSG or other flavourings, which are now under investigation for neurotoxicity.[86] These are not the only toxins present in SPI; there are also carcinogens such as nitrites.[87]

Perhaps the most pressing issue around soy consumption is that of endocrine disruption. Soy contains phytoestrogens which have been welcomed to protect from oestrogen excess and therefore oestrogen dependent cancers. The opposite might be true.[88]

To summarize, we can see that the ethical vegetarian has chosen an alternative which brings with it many problems. On the other hand, many foods consumed by meat-eaters are also undesirable. But the point I am trying to make here is that the ethical vegetarian is sacrificing her own health in order to spare animals from suffering. This sounds very much in line with the general Cancer miasm attitude we have discussed and I believe it to be a distinct feature of

85 Wallace, G.M. Studies on the Processing and Properties of Soymilk. Journal of Science and Food Agriculture 22:526-535, October 1971.

86 Blaylock RL. Excitotoxins, The Taste that Kills. Santa Fe. 1997. New Health Press

87 Rackis, et al. Evaluation of the Health Aspects of Soy Protein Isolates as Food Ingredients, prepared for FDA by Life Sciences Research Office, Federation of American Societies for Experimental Biology. 1979.

88 Petrakis, N.L. et al. Stimulatory influence of soy protein isolate on breast secretion in pre- and post-menopausal women. Cancer Epid. Bio. Prev. 1996; 5:785-794.
   Dees, C. et al. Dietary estrogens stimulate human breast cells to enter the cell cycle. Environmental Health Perspectives, 1997; 105(Suppl. 3):633-636.

this miasm. It is irrelevant whether a particular person in question is aware of the health problems of their diet or not; what is decisive here is that the person had to override their own natural inclination to eat the diet that they are evolutionary adapted to eat – in order to save another living being. The fact that many people do not succeed in suppressing their carnivorous instinct, should perhaps speak for itself.

With regards to the environment, a single individual cannot do much to change things for the better, leaving us feeling helpless and depressed. Becoming militant is not an option when you are in the Cancer miasm and a peaceful solution seems out of reach due to the interconnectedness of all issues and the sheer number of factors to consider. Again we see how an ideal goal cannot be attained. But because this goal is so vitally important for the survival of the species and the continuum of the planet, we are witness to our most enormous failure as a species and witness of our own self-destruction.

In spite of this sad reality, ethical vegetarians often try harder and harder to make a difference, but all they achieve is to seriously limit their own life. On top of this, their conscience suffers as they continuously feel guilty when they digress from their ideals even once in a while. Perfectionism and obsession ensues and we have shown how this can make a person sick. Unfortunately, there is no satisfactory answer to this problem and I will therefore close this issue with expressing my highest respect for the vegetarian ethical stance and my ultimate desire to find a way out of the dilemma.

Trust versus Control

As we left paradise, and with the dawn of self-consciousness, we developed angst. In turn we responded by leaving the state of "being" and entering the state of "doing". In the new age we have become very proficient at this to the extent that we have entered a state of "overdoing".

This means that because of our expanding knowledge in all fields we are now able to implement strategies and behaviours with the sole purpose of securing the future and eradicating anxiety once and for all. Everything we do, everything we study, everything we explore has the one aim – to reduce anxiety and make life safe and secure, with no pain, no accident, no risk to fear from tomorrow. Where an animal trusts, man controls.

For example, we control our children's education right from the start by enrolling them in a particular school at birth and subsequently shipping them from one activity to the next to provide enough "stimulation". This is because we are good parents, concerned and involved, but this is also because we do not trust that our child will find her own way. One of my patients recently stated "I still have not made any progress with teaching syllables to my daughter". The daughter is 3 years old. The same mother decided that her daughter was going to go to the best private secondary school for girls in the country when this daughter had just been born. Of course, if you have such intentions you cannot leave anything to chance, you must engage consciously to achieve this goal and this means you need to control pretty much everything in this child's life.

Is there a downside? Yes, because the child is not self-regulating or self-governed. Although, true to the Cancer attitude, all control is exerted with the best intentions, it is still harmful, because the child does not learn to use or harvest their own emotional intelligence which is one of two forces that govern human behaviour. In fact, most children and subsequently adults will (occasionally) notice a discrepancy between what they are asked to do and what they want to do, and of course this is normal. But when it reaches extremes, as in our society, a lot of compensatory behaviour will be necessary to numb any negative feelings that come up when we do not lead our lives in a self-governed way.

A simple example of this is that of a young mother who suddenly finds herself robbed of any freedom. Nobody could have prepared her for the relentless attention seeking of her new charge. It is very common for new mothers to hit the bottle (of wine) every evening once their child has been successfully settled. This is classic compensatory behaviour which will have serious consequences. Often a few glasses of wine are not enough; in many cases frequent chocolate consumption and that of other treats accompanies a seriously suffering diet as there is suddenly no time or energy to prepare a decent meal for herself. Combined with sleep deprivation and heavy demands on the physical body due to breastfeeding, this is a recipe for mental and emotional problems arising in due course. Considering this, it is surprising anyone manages to have more than one child. But they do, and this brings me onto another consequence of loss of trust.

Medical science has helped us to conquer acute disease and this is wonderful progress. It means that the days of fear of death from epidemics are over. In particular we do not need to worry about deadly childhood diseases such as scarlet fever, polio and diphtheria. My grandmother was full of stories about cousins dying and aunts losing more than half of their children from typhoid and other terrifying fevers. We also need not worry too much about death after accidents as emergency medical treatments are extremely efficient and successful (on the other hand we have more exposure to death from accidents due to inventions of cars, aeroplanes and motorcycles, etc).

However, in this modern age, when it comes to medicine, we see a shift from trust to doing to overdoing, i.e. control. In many instances we prevent instead of treat when indicated and this means we try to insure against a possible outcome. We see this dynamic at work in the practice of vaccination and in preventative blanket antibiotics for domesticated animals and in humans during operations and births. We are trying to prevent something we are terrified of, but cannot be even 50% sure it will happen. We have lost all trust that our bodies can defend and heal themselves without our intervention. The problem with this is not the attitude itself, but the compensatory behaviour. Vaccinations as a compensatory behaviour to insure against consequences of acute illness bring with it many negative aspects. Some of these are the carcinogenic or neurotoxic vaccine ingredients (such as formaldehyde and mercury), others become apparent over time, as the vaccinated body becomes less able to stage an acute reaction and shifts its immune reactions towards the chronic allergy and inflammation picture. Most of the evidence is clinical and many homeopaths are aware of these problems and so I will not discuss this any further. But the important point to remember is that the problems we cause are more wide-spread and less obvious than the problems we are trying to prevent. On the one hand, vaccination tries to prevent the death of a number of children, on the other hand it causes unnecessary suffering to all others who would not have needed the vaccination in the first place. These children become victims in the long run (unknowingly), when their metabolism and immune system become impaired and slip into chronic disease states. These disease states are much harder to manage and harder to cure with conventional medicine than the acute disease we tried to prevent by the vaccination.

When we look at acute illness, we see an enormous loss of trust in our innate and acquired immunity. Instead of trusting that the body of our child has evolved perfectly to handle a normal childhood fever, we fear the worst and use medication, i.e. Calpol/Paracetamol and antibiotics to handle a fever or infection. We are so removed from nature and understanding its natural processes that we can neither read nor intelligently manage natural processes in our child's bodies. When this happens only once, not much harm is done, but when it becomes routine to such an extent that we use these medical crotches at the first sign of anything untoward, we are beginning to impair our children's natural processes. As with anything that is not utilized, these become weak and eventually give up completely. We see this in our muscles, our mental capacities and our senses, but we refuse to recognise it in our immunity. One reason for this reluctance is of course the perceived danger and the anxiety of the affected person or parent. The other reason is the fact that we have the knowledge and means to manage acute disease with pharmaceuticals. So because we can, we do.

We also do this in another far more insidious and dangerous scenario: because we have Calpol at home we use it to sedate our children, even when we are not sure whether their pain is physical or emotional. I know of numerous parents who use Calpol routinely when their child cries at bedtime and cannot be settled. They tell themselves that if their child is crying, he must be in some sort of pain and so they feel justified in using Calpol. But children cry for many reasons including separation anxiety and manipulation. And most parents will know this deep down, but not admit it to themselves.

Actually, this practice enables many women to have several children close together. Why? Because it allows them to ensure peaceful nights at all times and peaceful days (no teething pains, no crying from headaches, tummy aches, ear aches, etc) Children, especially babies in their first year of life, are ill a lot and they need to be in order to acquire strong immunity. But all that crying, fussy behaviour and all those sleepless nights when baby is ill makes life very difficult, if not impossible, for a mother with several children and so Calpol is a welcome drug that makes having children much easier in this respect.

Calpol is not indicated, and entirely the wrong thing, to give when a child is crying.[89] It physically sedates the child and teaches them that a "drug" is appropriate when they are emotionally upset. I know of babies who, before they can speak even a single word, know how to point at

---

89 Of course, if a child is in unbearable pain, we need to relieve this pain as much and as soon as possible. Calpol is indicated at such times, if no other way is available. We also have homeopathy to relieve pain and it works in many cases. The problem is that most people do not know about it or do not trust it.

the Calpol bottle as soon as they are uncomfortable. This means that they have made the association of comfort with pharmaceuticals, a dangerous connection, you will agree.

Further, the question comes to mind how we will deal with a rebelling teen? It seems possible that an adolescent used to being given a sedative for every headache and growing pain has never learnt to ride out a relatively minor problem. He has never had the chance of trusting that it will resolve by itself within hours. And so it might be likely he will reach for recreational drugs, cigarettes and alcohol to help him through emotionally vulnerable times whenever it seems necessary. Don't we all remember those socially uncomfortable and embarrassing situations at that age? The times we wanted to impress, fit in, be noticed, be cool etc? My worry is that a child used to being sedated will turn into a teen sedating himself.

Back to Calpol/Paractamol, this drug has side-effects. One of these is a manifold increased risk of developing asthma and hay fever in later childhood.[90] Is a night of peace worth the risk of pushing your child into the chronic allergic picture?

We handle the more difficult and disharmonic side of having children with behaviours that numb or cover up the problem, but cause more trouble later on. We do this because we desire ease, harmony and peace at all times. We are truly children of Cancer and we are causing our own downfall. Because we refuse to recognise this mechanism at work, we observe helplessly but without guilt

---

90 Farquhar H, et al. The role of paracetamol in the pathogenesis of asthma. Clin Exp Allergy; 2010 Jan; 40(1):32-41.
   Eyers S, et al. Paracetamol in pregnancy and the risk of wheezing in offspring: a systematic review and meta-analysis. Clin Exp Allergy; 2011 Apr; 41(4):482-9

how our child's body deteriorates and becomes reliant on pharmaceuticals.

The fact is that the more we try to prevent a negative outcome, the more we may cause other, even worse outcomes. It may be that to a great extent, the widespread breakdown of immunity (allergies, HIV, cancer), healthy energy (ME states) and normal metabolism (diabetes) we see in the new age, is partially due to an "overdoing", i.e. a massive effort to control our medical future.

Disease in the Realm of Cancer

We have explored susceptibility and stimuli that marry to bring about the Cancer miasm. Let us now look at the type of physiological problem that is brought about by Cancer.

Syphilis moved the body into self-destruct mode. The disease spread to the heart, the brain and to the immune system as a whole, causing auto-immune conditions, mediated by a lack of cortisol output due to adrenal fatigue. Inflammation was also widespread and body parts were not only functioning poorly, but actually being destroyed in their physical structure. The self-healing capacity was greatly diminished due to inflammatory processes which remained unchecked by impaired immune responses. How could it get any worse?

Actually, it could.

With the advent of Cancer, we are now looking at functional and structural pathology that is due to alterations in DNA expression. This had so far not happened on such a grand scale. Let me explain.

Once we had learnt to remove some symptoms of Syphilis with mercury, arsenic and other, more modern drugs, we were still left with Syphilitic susceptibility and Syphilitic disease stimuli. But these were not able to bring about Syphilitic problems as those routes were blocked by treatments.

In addition, just as the body spared the adrenal glands from complete destruction during Syphilis, it now protects what is left of the thyroid, the brain, the heart and all the other places affected by Syphilis and mercury. It is our saving grace that the body is always self-preserving and will always try to stay alive by spreading the damage evenly. We could see it as a kind of osmosis of disease, seeping between compartments until all are saturated evenly.

In the Cancer miasm, there was no place left but the very core of the organism, i.e. the governing force and structures that had so far been spared. The place where decisions are made about how the organism functions are not brain and heart, but our DNA. We have two types of DNA and most of us homeopaths are not aware of this. We have DNA in the nucleus of every cell and we also have DNA in each mitochondrium.

A point of interest: Nuclear DNA is inherited equally from mother and father, but mitochondrial DNA (mDNA) is primarily inherited from the mother.[91] Perhaps it follows that the constitutional health of the mother is therefore of far greater importance than that of the father. Add 9 months of gestation in the mother's body and several months if not years of breastfeeding, should we not behave more responsibly before and during our fertile years?

---

91 Willner C. Oxidation-reduction Imbalances. Functional medicine, ch 21, p265ff, The institute for functional medicine; 2005

Mitochondria produce energy; they are the organelles which finish off the synthesis of ATP from glucose, fats and proteins. ATP is our energy currency, because ATP fuels chemical reactions. Since every single cell needs ATP continuously, we need a lot of it at all times for growth, maintenance, repair, movement, thought, reproduction, digestion, elimination, detoxification, immune defence, for our five senses and our nervous system. If our ATP levels are reduced, every function in our body becomes slower, less efficient and poorer quality. Therefore, if our mDNA is structurally or functionally damaged, other parts of our body will follow suit. It is just a matter of time. The classic example of mDNA damage and /or mitochondrial dysfunction is ME or Chronic Fatigue, but also fibromyalgia and other unexplained chronic pains.[92]

Mononucleosis, or glandular fever (GF), is often the acute illness that leaves ME in its wake. It is triggered by infection with the Epstein-Barr virus (EPV). This virus belongs to the herpes family and can remain latent for many years. Similarly to Human papilloma Virus (HPV), EPV also produces several types of cancer and this may happen after the virus has been latent in several types of immune cells for a potentially long time.

Thus homeopaths have good reason to place the acute disease glandular fever as well as the chronic version ME in the Cancer miasm.

The obvious disease process happening in the Cancer miasm is cancer. Cancer comes about when oncogenes are

---

92 Lapp CW, Cheyney PR, Rest J, et al. the chronic fatigue syndrome. Ann Int Med. 1995; 123(1):74-76
   Bland JS. Bioenergetics, Mitochondrial Function and Oxidative Stress in Functional Medicine. Functional Medicine, ch 30, p 501ff

activated[93] and tumour suppressor genes are inactivated. These genes reside in our DNA and we all have both of these. The good news is that for most of us and for most of our lives, the balance is in favour of life, not death.

There is consensus amongst scientists that reasons or causes for activation of cancer are not entirely known, but there is also consensus that some agents or causes are highly likely to have the above described effect on our DNA.

The International Agency for Research on Cancer (IARC) as part of the WHO publishes a list of carcinogenic agents[94]. This list is very long and contains some surprises, such as Tamoxifen (given to breast-cancer patients) and HRT/ the contraceptive pill. Other common substances include formaldehyde (ingredient of vaccines) and ethanol in alcoholic beverages. The IARC lists only substances which have been linked to cancer by published research and we can be sure that vested interests will try and keep this list as short as possible. For the same reason we can also be sure that we see only the tip of the iceberg.[95] Without wanting to sound too pessimistic, there is probably no man-made chemical that is not detrimental to our health in some way.[96] It has been estimated that since World War II 80,000 xenobiotic

---

93 More precisely: we all have healthy pre-oncogenes that are responsible for differentiated cell multiplication. In cancer, triggers cause mutation to change these genes into oncogenes which promotes unchecked cell proliferation without differentiation. The result is a growing mass of cells (tumour) that contains only one type of cell. This mass of cells does not perform any physiologically useful function and crowds out other useful cells

94 http://monographs.iarc.fr/ENG/Classification/ClassificationsAlphaOrder.pdf; 17th Jan 2012

95 Cohn BS, Wolff MS, Cirillo PM, and Sholtz RI. DDT and Breast Cancer in Young Women: New data on the significance of age at exposure. Environm health Perspct, 2007; 115910:1406-14

96 Sanborn M, Cole D, Kerr K, et al. Systematic Review of pesticide human health effects. Ontario College of family Physicians. 2004; 1-186.

substances have been introduced into the environment.[97] A xenobiotic is defined as a chemical substance that is foreign, and usually harmful, to living organisms[98]. Perhaps xenobiotics are not all carcinogenic, but they may produce poor energy states or other problems that in a roundabout way will increase the risk of cancer anyway. This leaves us with a very poor outlook indeed, because there is almost no escape from toxic exposure. All we can do is minimise it and hope that we can strengthen our body with beneficial substances and therapies to avoid the worst case scenario.

On the same pessimistic note, every year more and more cases of inheritable and actually inherited mutations to cancer genes are found in cancer patients. This means that the incidence of inherited active oncogenes and inactive tumour suppressor genes is increasing, sadly supporting our miasmatic theory.

The realisation that carcinogenic substances are omnipresent somehow resonates with the character of the disease. Cancer can happen in any part of our body, even in liquids such as lymph and blood. It can also move and recur once it has been removed. The omnipresence of toxins and the ability of cancer to strike anywhere and anytime also resonates with the globalisation (well-connectedness) stage of social evolution as explained above. It is as if the dominant attitude of society is reflected in the diseases the society produces.

Another example for the character of disease reflecting a dominant attitude in society is diabetes mellitus. This disease, whether type 1 or 2, involves a life-threatening

97 Shea KM. protecting our children from environmental hazards in the face of limited data-a precautionary approach is needed. J Pediatr. 2004; 145: 153-56

98 Webster's New World Dictionary of American English, 3rd College edition.

problem with blood sugar balance. I repeat: the problem is essentially one of too much sugar in the blood and the body struggling to find a healthy balance. And here is the parallel – the main susceptibility for the Cancer miasm is the need for harmony and peace after the extreme seesaw of Syphilis. We needed to find a balance, a sustainable plateau somewhere on middle ground. Our society is striving towards this balance with attitudes of tolerance and harmony, but since this is difficult to achieve we compensate with substances that cause blood sugar problems such as sugar, alcohol, stimulants and drugs. In a nutshell – we want emotional balance but we achieve blood sugar imbalance. Of course there is nothing wrong with the desire for balance, actually it is a very good idea, but this balance could be found naturally and in a healthy way. (More about that later.)

In all cases of type 1 and in many cases of type 2, life needs to be sustained by pharmaceuticals. It is not only that a dangerous rise (or fall) in blood sugar can lead to instant death, but also the fact that severe collateral damage can be expected in other organs such as the kidneys and peripheral circulation which make this condition a serious problem.

Diabetes type 2, or adult onset diabetes, has so far not convincingly been linked to altered gene expression. Even in the eyes of conventional medicine it is mostly a life-style and dietary problem and this view is of course supported by everything we have said so far. In diabetes type 2, blood sugar problems come about because body cells do not react to insulin. This means that any sugar circulating in the blood cannot be removed from it, and piles up until it becomes dangerously high and leads to coma, then death. There are many theories why this sensitivity to insulin may be lost in some people, and they involve a combination of factors including exposure to environmental pollution,[99] lack of exercise and poor mineral supply (as certain minerals such as chromium and zinc are needed for the transport of sugar into cells). In a cereal based diet the minerals in question are in poor supply and the heavy consumption of plain white sugar and alcohol, so common in the new age, increases this deficit even further. This is because the digestion of sugar and metabolic clearance of alcohol need these very minerals that we are deficient in. Eating plain white sugar (and brown sugar is not much better) and drinking alcohol therefore presents us with a double whammy. It does not supply us with anything and it robs us of even more. We are back to our initial argument that poor diet and unfavourable lifestyle can bring about serious disease.[100]

Luckily for some, insulin sensitivity is lost by degrees over many years. As long as it is just a mild reduction in sensitivity it is possible to manage (and perhaps cure) it by

---

99 Lee DH et al. Associations between serum concentrations of persistent organic pollutants and insulin resistance among nondiabetic adults: results from the National Health and Nutrition Examination Survey 1999-2002. Diabetes Care, 2007; 30(3):622-8

100 Kant AK. Consumption of energy-dense, nutrient-poor foods by adult Americans: nutritional and health implications. The third national health and nutrition examination survey, 1988-1994. AmJ Clin Nutr. 2000; 72:929-36

Ames BN, Wakimoto P. Are vitamin and mineral deficiencies a major cancer risk? Nat.Rev Cancer. 2002; 2:694-704

Hung HC, Joshipura KJ, et al. Fruit and vegetable intake and risk of major chronic disease. J Natl Cancer Inst. 2004; 96:1577-84

Blount BC, Mack MM, et al. Folate deficiency causes uracil misincorporation into human DNA and chromosome breakage:implications for cancer and neuronal damage. Proc Natl Acad Sci U S A. 1997; 94:3290-95

Kim,YI. Folate and carcinogenesis: evidence, mechanisms and implications. J Nutri Biochem. 1999; 10:66-88

diet and lifestyle measures alone. From an attitude point of view, diabetes type 2 is very much a problem of poor discipline and excess and so is definitely strongly Sycotic. But because it involves a major homeostatic mechanism (back to the issue of finding balance) and because it can be fatal within hours, I would place it in the Cancer miasm.

Diabetes type 1 does involve alteration of gene expression quite similar to cancer. The altered gene expression is acquired[101], i.e. triggered by unknown substances, although the risk of developing diabetes type1 is higher in people who have relatives with the same disease, suggesting an inherited component. Scientists speculate about a virus or other infection being a trigger of acquired type1. Once triggered it takes 5 to 10 years for the pancreatic insulin-producing cells to be completely destroyed by T-cells.

A very interesting fact is that diabetes type 1 involves in some variants an additional autoimmune reaction against insulin (not only pancreatic insulin-producing cells). And here is the surprise – it has been discovered that insulin is also produced in the thymus gland. Researchers believe that the proximity of insulin to maturing T-cells might give some protection against auto-immune attacks by T-cells on healthy tissue and therefore against development of diabetes type 1.

As homeopaths we hold the thymus gland in high esteem, because it is the seat of maturation of immune cells. It has been scientifically established that some of these cells also protect against cancer and auto-immunity. Many Homeopaths believe that the thymus gland becomes damaged

---

101 Knip, M., Veijola, R. et al. Environmental Triggers and Determinants of Type 1 Diabetes. Diabetes 54. 2005; S125–S136.

through childhood vaccinations, but we have no proof of this. If this were so, then any auto-immune disease, but especially diabetes type 1, could be linked to vaccinations, at least in part.

Auto-immunity

All auto-immune diseases are Syphilitic, because they involve the body destroying itself. From my point of view, some auto-immune diseases are also part of the Cancer picture and I would place them here as soon as they affect homeostatic control systems in our body. This denotes the above mentioned problem with "balance". Examples of auto-immune diseases that are in the Cancer miasm as well as in the Syphilitic miasm are, therefore: *Hashimoto's* (affecting the metabolic rate via the thyroid gland) and *diabetes type 1* (affecting the balance of blood sugar via the pancreas), and there may be more. All other auto-immune problems not involving homeostatic systems such as Crohn's, psoriasis, MS and Lupus are just plain Syphilitic (as if this were not bad enough).

There is another aspect to auto-immunity that we have touched on above. In recent years it has become apparent that more and more people react negatively to eating wheat, in particular gluten, a protein in wheat. It has been scientifically established that similarly to oncogenes and insulin genes we have genes to do with tolerance of gluten (and some suspect cereals in general). We know that in coeliacs these genes express the no-tolerance stance. There is a new school of thought that is investigating the possibility, or even probability, of many if not most people with auto-immunity (about 70%) to have these genes set to no-tolerance.

The mechanism by which a no-tolerance to gluten would bring the immune system to attack own body cells is not understood, but there are several theories. The most plausible one seems to be the idea of intestinal permeability linked to cellular mimicry.

This goes as follows:

An unknown trigger has set cereal tolerance genes to no-tolerance (possibly in past generations). Cereals arriving in the intestines cause inflammation and a loosening of "tight junctions" (the name for gaps between cells in the gut lining). Through these, partially digested cereal-derived gluten particles (and others) enter lymphatic tissue blood stream[102]. Gluten is a protein and as such is made up of amino acid sequences, a type of code. Because of the no-tolerance setting, immune cells are programmed to destroy anything with this particular amino acid code. The body's own cells have protein markers on their outside surface, dangling into the extracellular fluid, so to speak. These markers may contain a similar sequence of amino acids to gluten particle codes. The immune cells set to destroy the gluten code will also target anything they pass by that looks similar. This may be a thyroid cell, or a pancreas cell. Or indeed any cell. Once the auto-immune cells are active they remain so for MONTHS, even without subsequent exposure to cereal derived particles. And the amount of gluten the

---

[102] Lammers KM, Lu R, Brownley J, et al. Gliadin induces an increase in intestinal permeability and zonulin release by binding to the chemokine receptor CXCR3. July 2008; Gastroenterology 135 (1): 194–204.

Assimakopoulos SF, Papageorgiou I, Charonis A. Enterocytes' tight junctions: From molecules to diseases. World J Gastrointest Pathophysiol. 2011 Dec 15; 2(6): 123-37

size of a pea is enough to set the auto-immune cascade into motion.

Food for Thought

While many individual AI (autoimmune) diseases are rare, collectively they are thought to affect approximately 8 per cent of the US population – 24 million persons. (NIH. Autoimmune Diseases Coordinating Comm. Autoimmune Diseases Research Plan. 2006)

Autoimmune disorders occur 10 times more commonly in coeliac disease (CD) than in the general population (CMLS; Cell, Mol. Life Sci. 62, 2005; 7791-799)

The most frequent reported associations (with gluten intolerance) are with type 1 diabetes mellitus and auto-immune thyroiditis. (Autoimmunity Reviews 6, 2007; 559-565)

Patients with CD are at risk for developing thyroid disease, with an overall 3-fold higher frequency than in controls. (Amer.J.Gastro. 2001; Vol.96, No.3)

For every symptomatic patient with CD there are 8 patients with CD that have no GI symptoms. (Gastroenterology 2001; 120: 636-651)

Originally considered a rare malabsorption syndrome of childhood, CD is now recognised as a common condition that may be diagnosed at any age and may affect many organ systems. (NEJM; 357; 17 Oct 25, 2007)

Most patients who present with neurological manifestations of gluten sensitivity have no GI symptoms. (Lancet Neurol 2010; 9; 318-30)

...every time the disease (CD) is diagnosed in an adult, that person has for decades had disease in a latent or silent stage... (N Engl J Med Oct.23, 2003; 1673-4)

Cardiovascular disease was the most common cause of death in CD, followed by malignancy (JAMA, Sept.16, 2009; Vol.302, No.11)

Autoimmune diseases are the third leading cause of morbidity and mortality in the industrialised world, surpassed only by cancer and heart disease. (The Journal of Immunology, 2005; 175: 4119-4126)

It may be possible that all auto-immune disease states are partially due to a non-tolerance of gluten, or indeed other items in our diet that should not be there. We already discussed lectins under Psora and the dairy intolerance gene under Tuberculosis. The selection of tissues to be destroyed by auto-immune cells seems to be random, but homeopaths might say that it depends on the susceptibility. Generally speaking, non-tolerance of gluten (and perhaps all cereals) can have devastating effects anywhere in the body.

And here is the most shocking news:

It is suspected that up to 50% of people of European descent have their cereal tolerance genes set to no-tolerance (or at least partial tolerance only, as there are several genes). There also seems to be a process of positive selection going on, so that the no-tolerance genes are becoming more prevalent.[103] This is opposing expectations which assumed that, in agricultural populations, negative selection would cause an increase in cereal tolerance.[104]

With this we have come full circle. What began 10,000 years ago with Psora has caught up with us and taken on a life of its own. In the age of Cancer we are dying a slow and cruel death from something we believe is good for us.

Toxic World – Toxic Body

We have extensively discussed the susceptibility and stimuli that come together and bring about the Cancer miasm.

---

[103] Rubio-Tapia et al.; Kyle, RA; et al. Increased Prevalence and Mortality in Undiagnosed Celiac Disease. Gastroenterology, 2009; 137 (1): 88–93.

[104] Catassi, C. Where Is Celiac Disease Coming From and Why?. Journal of Pediatric Gastroenterology & Nutrition. 2005; 03000

Zhernakova A et al. Evolutionary and Functional Analysis of Celiac Risk Loci Reveals SH2B3 as a Protective Factor against Bacterial Infection. 2010; The American Journal of Human Genetics.

This is because as homeopaths we must always satisfy the law which states that disease only comes about when susceptibility marries stimulus.

We have also shown that to a homeopath's great advantage, we have finally reached a point where science has caught up with us and is supporting our view. This may help us in spreading our message, as we do not need to use our at times alienating homeopathic terminology. We can use widely accepted and understood words and messages.

Whichever terminology we use, when we arrive at the Cancer miasm, as homeopaths we must change our perception dramatically and realise that the Kentian case analysis is really not sufficient and may be actually dangerous to the patient.

Let me explain.

If you stop a patient from being a door-mat, of being a perfectionist, of being an ethical vegetarian etc., he will not suddenly be cured of his Cancer miasm condition. You know that you have to remove all stimuli too. Will the patient magically become aware of individual stimuli? Or will many remain hidden from his perception or indeed his influence even with repeated mental/emotional prescriptions?

For example, most people are not aware, and never will be, that cereals may cause auto-immune disease and that dairy may cause cancer. They believe that it is good for them and so they will not remove it. If it is not part of your awareness that something is bad for you, how would you magically become aware of it with a homeopathic remedy?

In some cases and with regards to some stimuli it is possible, but most of the time probably not.

Similarly, knowing that electromagnetic radiation is carcinogenic does not help you to eliminate it from your environment and does not stop you from being exposed to it.

And so there are many stimuli that are carcinogenic, ie provoking diseases of the Cancer miasm that will not be identified and not removed for whatever reason. They will continue maintaining the patient's disease in spite of any remedies given (or the remedies will help only for a while).

"But" I can hear you saying "if I remove the susceptibility, I do not need to remove the stimuli. They won't have an effect anymore." This is a big error. Healing is not instant, it takes time to complete after a remedy has been given. In fact, before the healing has been completed by the vital force, the disease is continuously being triggered anew by the onslaught of stimuli in our toxic environment.

In addition to the problem of omnipresent environmental maintaining causes there is a new aspect that has entered our lives since the start of the Cancer miasm – in our modern world we are bombarded by carcinogenic substances beyond a tolerance level any human being can handle.

Our water, our air, our magnetic fields and our foods are poisoned. In addition, our living habits (sleep, exercise, light exposure, social interaction) are often unhealthy. Further, we have inherited weaknesses that make us ill at an earlier age, as our disease-causing genes have already been triggered by previous generations.

Toxicity Quotes and Statistics

US pesticide use is 4 billion pounds annually, that is 8 pounds for every person (Body Burden, Environmental Working Group, 2005)

Over 167 synthetic chemicals and carcinogens are now found in the average human body (US EPA National Adipose Tissue Survey, 1982)

The concentration of PBDEs (a flame retardant) in the breast milk of women inhabiting the remote Faroe islands has increased threefold between 1987 and 1999. (Fangstrom B, Strid A, et al. A retrospective study of PBDEs and PCBs in human milk from the Faroe Islands. Environ Health. 2005; 4(1);12)

Environmental agents, including chemical carcinogens, are modifiable risk factors to which over 70% of breast cancers have been attributed (DeBruin LS et al. Environ Health Perspect. 2002 Feb; 110 (Suppl 1):119-128)

The modern world is plagued with expanding epidemics of diseases related to metabolic dysfunction. The factors that are driving obesity, diabetes, cardiovascular disease, hypertension,, and dyslipidemias (collectively termed metabolic syndrome) are usually ascribed to a mismatch between the body's homeostatic nutrient requirements and dietary excess, coupled with insufficient exercise. The environmental obesogen hypothesis proposes that exposure to a toxic chemical burden is superimposed on these conditions to initiate or exacerbate the development of obesity and its associated health consequences. (Grun F, Blumberg B, Perturbed nuclear receptor signalling by environmental obesogens as emerging factors in the obestity crisis. Rev Endocr Metab Disord. 2007 Jun; 8(2):161-71)

You could say that the average human being living in a developed country has reached a toxic saturation level beyond which disease always ensues.

You could say that we are all so toxic that only one further drop is necessary to cause the tank to spill.

You could say that toxicity permeates every aspect of our life so that no escape is possible.

You could say that living as an individual in a society that as a whole supports the Cancer miasm, you will be affected whether you are individually susceptible or not.

Cancer, the disease, affects any organ or system and Cancer, the miasm, affects every individual living in a society dominated by it.

The only way susceptibility comes into it, is in the degree and age of onset of your disease (and this is where therapies may be extremely beneficial).

So I would rather have diabetes type 2 than diabetes type 1, but I would rather have diabetes type 1 than cancer. I would choose Hashimoto's over ME, and I would prefer hay fever to nut allergy.

We are all going to be victims of the Cancer miasm. Any therapy, including homeopathy, can (only) buy us time and/or reduce the severity. In many cases, if conducted properly, this will be enough to lead a productive and healthy life for 70-80 years and only then descend into chronic disease. If not done properly, we will begin deteriorating much sooner.

Most of us love homeopathy and are drawn to it because we are victims of the Cancer miasm and love to believe humans are sick because they are unhappy. In other words, we believe Kent was right. Perhaps he was and still is right up to a point just as Newton was and still is right up to a point. But when you enter the 20th century realm of particles versus waves, Newton simply does not apply anymore. In the same way, Kent simply does not apply to Cancer.

The main therapeutic implication of this insight is that we cannot treat a disease of the Cancer miasm with the

Kentian method. The patient is not sick because he is unhappy, he is sick because he is drowning in disease-provoking agents.

The Benefits of the Cancer Miasm

Cancer, the miasm, is not all bad. Just as with the other miasms, this new miasm saved humanity from extinction. Putting aside disharmony, conflict, apartheid, racism, sexism and dogma, and striving for tolerance, kindness, acceptance, harmony and peace is a wonderful development. Nobody in their right mind would choose to go back to Syphilitic dogma and cruelty just because we are now seeing an explosion in chronic disease at an early age. Even if we have to put up with deep and incurable disease in our children, we would much rather prefer to be ill than to be tortured. This is because the new age has also brought us enough science to make illness bearable and in many cases almost unnoticeable. So we are not really making any great concessions.

The real benefits of the age of Cancer, however, have (for various reasons, usually to do with greed and arrogance) not yet been realised to their full potential:

>   Through science and globalisation we now have at hand enough knowledge to treat acute and chronic disease successfully, at least so that most of us can hope to live for 70 or 80 years without medication and/or pain. Various alternative medicine disciplines would achieve this in concert with conventional medicine.

>   We also have at hand ways of harvesting and using energy that does not pollute the environment.

> We know many ways of food production and storage that do not harm the soil and do not pollute the environment or the people and animals eating the food.

> We have organic animal husbandry; organic farming methods and sustainable fishing can easily be implemented.

> There is no need to pollute the oceans, rivers, lakes or the water table.

> We have humane and healthy ways of birth control so we could, if we were reasonable, reduce the world's population to a sustainable size.

For most problems of a global nature we have answers. And these answers were found because we were able to scientifically explore the planet, its organic and inorganic life.

So let us thank the Cancer miasm for advancing us, but let us make use of our newly found knowledge and wisdom to realise our potential.

Conclusion

The journey of humanity from cave to computer was necessary and inevitable once set in motion. At each step on the way we chose the most advantageous option for society as a whole. There never was an alternative and a return was impossible. Onwards and upwards we strived through the ages. There is no doubt that social evolution was beneficial for the species as it ensured its survival. Paradoxically, the more certain the survival of the species became, the more the individual's health suffered.

With regards to our discussion of chronic disease, one major purpose of this book was to show how susceptibility does nothing without stimulus. Following on from this, we identified many stimuli which many homeopaths would not dare consider. Our journey through the ages from cave to computer has shown us in detail those major stimuli we oversee in the treatment of our patients.

Of course we are still homeopaths and we still adhere to our theory and practice. We employ our strategies to reduce the predisposition to be affected by particular stimuli. As the patient goes through life, this is immensely helpful, as he becomes more resistant.

This idea is easy to understand when we take susceptibility to infection as an example. But what about the predisposition for developing chronic disease? Can we really treat this with homeopathy?

Maintaining Causes

There are two types of maintaining cause and this is most important for us to understand, because this is where homeopaths can go wrong.

There is the obvious type of smoking and drinking too much alcohol, living in a damp building or never going outdoors. These behaviours are obviously not good for anyone, regardless of susceptibility. Susceptibility only determines how much of this wrong behaviour we can handle; it sets our personal threshold, so to speak. So whereas smoking is bad for every human being, some can get away with it, because they are stronger for various reasons (known and unknown). Homeopathy may in some cases be used to increase the threshold of tolerance, but permanent success is only possible if the behaviour is stopped or if homeopathy is taken continuously alongside the disease-stimulating behaviour.

The second type of maintaining cause is of surprisingly similar nature, the difference being that this type comprises of behaviours/substances that are commonly accepted as fit for human consumption or indeed even seen as health-building.

Just as with the first type, we are talking about behaviours/substances which are detrimental to any member of the human species. The only difference susceptibility makes is in the degree in which these affect us. Please be aware that they definitely affect everyone negatively, simply because humans have not evolved to handle them.

Our discussion of human social evolution has shown us what these maintaining causes are: cereals, dairy, pulses (including soy), yeasts, processed sugar, processed fats, mercury, arsenic, any synthetically produced chemical entering our body via food, drink, water, air and pharmaceuticals, and finally radiation.

In a nutshell, it is my view that this has made gluten, dairy, sugar and yeast exposure a miasmatic stimulus for respectively developing Psora, Tuberculosis and Sycosis. Syphilis is mainly the concoction of the previous topped up with mercury and Cancer throws in synthetic toxins to finish us off completely.

There were many other factors playing their part on each level, but these dietary changes and their consequences played an important part.

Homeopathy may be able to raise the tolerance threshold to these substances, but again only if it is used continuously alongside the consumption or exposure. It is my view that any "cure" we see in our patients is nothing but a truce. And this truce can be of literally any length depending on the totality of behaviours the patients engages in and the totality of substances the patients is exposed to. Part of our treatments must be to explain this to the patient, so as to help him take responsibility for his own health.

Therapeutic Implications

For me the facts are clear. Chronic disease is to a large degree triggered by wrong life-style choices. These are often compensatory behaviours that are supposed to help us bear the brunt of human existence. Whilst it is extremely important to become aware of those parts of our lives we find unbearable, and whilst it is important to find ways to make them more bearable, we also must stop drowning our sorrows and numbing our fears, because the substances and behaviours we use make us sick.

When we are prepared to do this for several months at a time and then for the rest of our lives, even if it seems hard work at first, we may find that much of our physical and emotional, as well as mental, unhappiness simply dissolves into thin air. This is because many health problems are just a result of wrong living. And by that I mean unsuitable for homo sapiens per se. No exceptions.

What about the original susceptibility to chronic disease, the fact that we are human and self-aware? Will we ever conquer this?

Probably not. This makes it all the more important to give this susceptibility as little as possible to feed on. With all our miasmatic inheritance on our backs, and with all the Sycotic temptation around us, we will have to be dedicated and watchful if we want to remain healthy and happy into old age.

The truth of the matter is that we have all left paradise.

Nevertheless it is possible to find our way back not by losing self-awareness and becoming animals again, but by transcending anxiety with reason. The quest we began with Psora, we may successfully conclude with Cancer.

A Cure

When we left nature we acquired anxiety. Subsequently we were lost in a wilderness of emotional anxiety, mental drudge and physical peril. Our consciousness did not permit us to trust that we would be taken care of on any level. Even spirituality did not help sufficiently.

Now, after our epic journey, we have come full circle and we are in the position to re-enter a state of trust. Whereas before Psora this trust was instinctual, now, thanks to Cancer, it is based on reason. And reason has two parts to it – scientific knowledge and emotional intelligence.

We have sufficient knowledge and experience to resolve mankind's most pressing reasons to be anxious. We are able to look after our bodies, our emotions and our minds. We are able to look after the earth, the oceans and the skies. We are able to look after the parts without harming the whole.

When we have a moment to sit back and reflect, we should realise that nowadays there should be nothing to worry about.

Of course, we have not implemented all our knowledge and wisdom yet, but as more and more people complete their personal journey from cave to computer, a critical mass of people will push open the gates to a world where there is enough for everyone and where everybody is good enough.

Appendix 1 — Cancer & Science

Alternative medicine is not alone in its belief that chronic disease can to a large part be prevented by life-style measures. The following article shows how science and conventional medicine are moving in the same direction. Interestingly, far from staying only with the most obvious life-style measures, my points about the collective attitude of a society and its behaviour as well as the issue of reaching a critical mass of people are also supported by the authors of the study cited.

"More Than Half of All Cancer Is Preventable, Experts Say"
ScienceDaily (Mar. 28, 2012)[105]

More than half of all cancer is preventable, and society has the knowledge to act on this information today, according to Washington University public health researchers at the Siteman Cancer Center in St. Louis.

In a review article published in Science Translational Medicine[106] the investigators outline obstacles they say stand in the way of making a huge dent in the cancer burden in the United States and around the world.

"We actually have an enormous amount of data about the causes and preventability of cancer," says epidemiologist Graham A. Colditz, MD, DrPH, the Niess-Gain Professor at the School of Medicine and associate director of prevention and control at the Siteman Cancer Center. "It's time we made an investment in implementing what we know."

---

[105] http://www.sciencedaily.com/releases/2012/03/120328154433.htm, accessed on 21st August 2012

[106] Colditz GA, Wolin KY, Gehlert S. Applying What We Know to Accelerate Cancer Prevention. Sci Transl Med 28 March 2012: Vol. 4, Issue 127, p. 127rv4

What we know, according to Colditz and his co-authors, is that lifestyle choices people make and that society can influence in a number of ways – from tobacco use to diet and exercise – play a significant role in causing cancer. Specifically, the researchers cite data demonstrating that smoking alone is responsible for a third of all cancer cases in the United States. Excess body weight and obesity account for another 20 percent.

But beyond individual habits, they argue that the structure of society itself – from medical research funding to building design and food subsidies – influences the extent of the cancer burden and can be changed to reduce it.

The obstacles they see to implementing broad cancer prevention strategies are:

> Skepticism that cancer can be prevented. Smoking rates in different states demonstrate that 75 percent of lung cancer in the United States could be prevented with elimination of cigarette smoking.

> The short-term focus of cancer research. Benefits of prevention may be underestimated because they take decades to show up, and research funding often spans five years or less.

> Intervening too late in life to prevent cancer. Strategies like vaccination against cancer-causing viruses, such as the human papilloma virus that causes cervical cancer, work best when begun early, in this case before young people begin sexual activity.

> Research focuses on treatment, not prevention. Treatments focus only on a single organ after diagnosis but behavioral changes reduce cancer and death rates from many chronic diseases.

> Debate among scientists. They say health experts have a moral responsibility to highlight cancer risk factors even without knowing the biological mechanism by which they cause cancer.
> Societal factors that affect health. Tobacco policy and government subsidies don't do enough to discourage unhealthy behavior, and in some cases they make the unhealthy options more accessible, especially in low-income communities.
> Lack of collaboration across disciplines. Scientists and health experts must work together to learn what causes cancer, communicate that to the public and work with community leaders to implement policies that help people lead healthier lives, they say.
> The complexity of implementing broad changes. With so many players involved, from health-care providers to government regulators to individuals, it will be difficult to implement broad change over the long term.

According to the American Cancer Society, an estimated 1,638,910 new cancer cases will be diagnosed this year in the United States. Also this year, 577,190 Americans are expected to die of cancer. Only heart disease kills more people in this country. And Colditz's research has shown that these cancer prevention strategies would reduce the burden of heart disease and other chronic conditions as well.

Despite the obstacles, Colditz and his colleagues point to some successes that they say demonstrate that broad change is possible. One example is the relatively quick elimination of unhealthy trans fats from the national diet. And the National Cancer Institute (NCI) has reported that lung cancer rates are declining in both men and women, supporting the benefits of tighter tobacco control policy.

"After working in public health for 25 years, I've learned that if we want to change health, we need to change policy," says co-author Sarah J. Gehlert, PhD, the E. Desmond Lee Professor of Racial and Ethnic Diversity at the Brown School of Social Work and the School of Medicine. "Stricter tobacco policy is a good example. But we can't make policy change on our own. We can tell the story, but it requires a critical mass of people to talk more forcefully about the need for change."

Appendix 2 — Practical Advice

The ideal diet for human beings, regardless of race or tradition is the Paleo diet or hunter-gatherer diet. It needs to be done correctly to work. This means every meal must consist of 75% vegetables with 25% animal protein. A few pieces of fruit are also suitable, but never to the exclusion of vegetables. The second requirement for this diet to work is that sufficient aerobic exercise needs to be engaged in, and this translates to at least 3hrs strenuous endurance activity per week.

It is important not to eat fruit for breakfast because this stimulates an extraordinary insulin response and is therefore detrimental to blood sugar balance and the adrenal glands. I therefore would insist that vegetables are eaten even for breakfast.

It is obviously impossible for many people to go cold turkey and make changes overnight. It will also be impossible for many people to switch all lifestyle choices and behaviours to 100% positive. And, as things stand, we obviously cannot completely avoid toxic pollution.

This does not mean we should give up before we even started. We could educate everybody as to what the ideal case would be. Then, we should try to help them to move towards this scenario at their individual pace. Even a small change will have positive effects.

Whilst remaining compassionate and sympathetic at all times, we need to become aware of where and when we become enablers of negative behaviours. This is when homeopathy becomes an art, because practitioners need to become creative in their way of bringing the patient back to health.

Interestingly, the simillimum does not only apply to finding the remedy, it also applies to managing the patient.

Beyond this, my attitude to improving health has long been one of balance. I believe health can be likened to a bank account in that we can pay in credits and take out debits. The more we pay in the healthier we become. We can also take out debits, but only if we are in credit to start with! This concept makes life easy because it allows people to understand how much of their health is their own making. And it allows people to indulge occasionally without feeling guilty, because they know they are generally in credit.

After all I said in this book, I would still apply the 80/20 rule: 80% discipline alternating with 20% enjoyment. We do not live only to prevent disease in the future, we also live to enjoy the present. But in true Yin and Yang style, the present can best be enjoyed if the past and future are disciplined.

Bibliography

Blaylock RL. *Excitotoxins. The Taste that Kills.* Santa Fe, Health Press, 1997 – for the effects of MSG , aspartame and other flavourings on the nervous system.

Campbell-McBride N. *Gut and Psychology Syndrome.* Cambridge, Medinform Publishing, 2010 – gut flora link to allergy and mental disease

Cordain L. *The Paleo Diet.* Hoboken: John Wiley & Sons, 2002 – explores reasons for and effect of a hunter-gatherer diet.

D'Adamo P. *The Eat Right Diet.* London: Century, 1998 – Explains the author's theory of the blood type diet. My inspiration for the division into hunter, settler and nomad.

Diamond J. *Guns, Germs and Steel. A short history of everybody for the last 13,000 years.* London, Vintage (2005) – explores the reasons why history unfolded differently for different societies.

Fallon S, Enig MG. *Cinderella's Dark Side.* Nexus magazine, 2000 Vol 7, no 3 – discusses the soy issue; many references.

Institute for Functional Medicine. *Textbook of Functional Medicine.* Gig Harbour, 2005 – excellent textbook of integrated medicine; for exploring dysfunctions of the human organism in holistic fashion; dysfunctions are seen as result of lifelong interactions among environment, lifestyle and genetic disposition; current on scientific data, physiology and pathology.

Montefiore SS. *Jerusalem, The Biography.* London, Phoenix, 2011 – 3,000 years of Middle Eastern History, at times raging Sycosis/Syphilis; clash of monotheistic Israelites with other early urban societies; terrific account of the Temple siege.

Wilson JL. *Adrenal Fatigue, The 21st Century Stress Syndrome.* Petaluma, Smart Publications, 2001 – explains cause and effect of adrenal insufficiency.